Moisés Asís

ABRIDGED APITHERAPY 101 CLINICAL FORMS

Asís, Moisés. *Abridged Apitherapy 101 clinical forms*. 160 pp. [This is a black/white, English shorter edition with some Spanish entries, in comparison with full-color *Apitherapy 101 clinical forms / Formularios clínicos de Apiterapia 101*].

Library of Congress Control Number available upon request

Independently published

Available from Amazon.com and other bookstores

Author pictures in back cover and Chap.15: Dina Lílit Asís-Mendoza (Miami, USA)

Other pictures and diagrams are from the author's archive in *Apiterapia 101 para todos*, *Apitherapy 101 Clinical Forms / Formularios clínicos de Apiterapia 101*, *Acupuntura y hatha yoga para las disfunciones sexuales*, *Propóleo: el oro púrpura de las abejas*, *Apiterapia A-Bee-Z*, and other books; his pages in Facebook.com, Linkedin.com, **Facebook.com/Apitherapy101**, **Facebook.com/groups/BeesForLife WorldApitherapy**, and **Facebook.com/The-Open-International-University-for-Complementary-Medicines**; and from Bees for Life, **Pixabay.com**, **Pinterest.com**, **Shivambu.in**, and other authorized sources.

OTHER ACKNOWLEDGEMENTS: Thanks to my daughter Dina L. Asís-Mendoza and my wife Teresa Asís; and thanks for the comments or information from Miguel Abad, Karina Ángel, American Apitherapy Society, Apitherapy News, Marco Biagi, Bruno Burlando, Héctor Cielo, Laura Cornara, Antonio Couto, Deutscher Apitherapie Bund, Franco Feraboli, Alfredo C. Henríquez, Zachary Huang, Martín Juárez, Arunas Kulikauskas, Jonathan Lee, Homero Llerena, Sunil Munot, Eva Oriwall, Pedro Pérez, María I. Prado, Sociedad Mexicana de Apiterapia, Ştefan Stângaciu, Trinidad Terrazas, and Jianbo Xiao.

CONTENTS

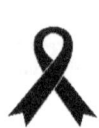
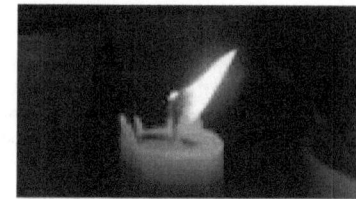

IN MEMORIAM

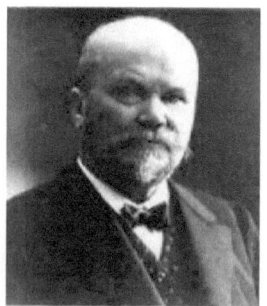

Filip Terč, MD, Czechia - Slovenia (1844 - 1917), Father of Modern Apitherapy.

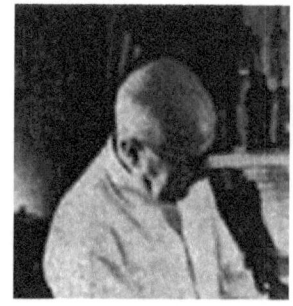

Bodog F. Beck, MD, Hungary - USA (1871 - 1942), Father of American Apitherapy.

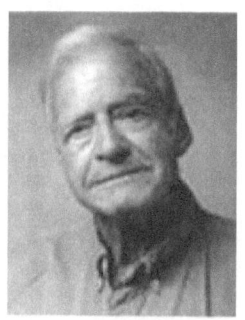

Charles Mraz, USA (1905 - 1999), American Apitherapy pioneer and promotor.

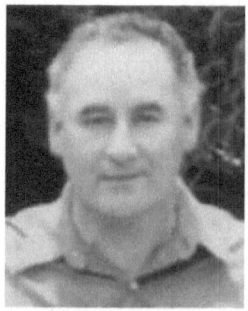

Fernando López Hernández, MD, Mexico (1955 - 2001), Apitherapy promotor in Latin America.

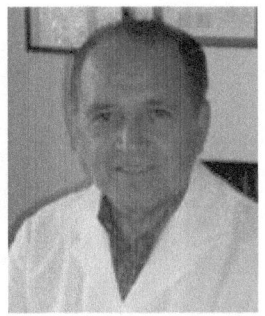

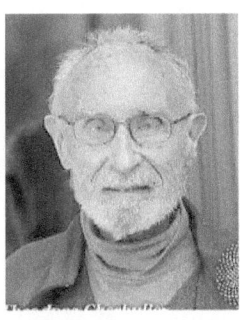

Vicente A. Ferrer Candia, ScD, Chile (1945 - 2007), Apitherapy promotor in Latin America.

Théodore Cherbuliez, MD, Switzerland - USA (1927 - 2016), Worldwide Apitherapy promotor.

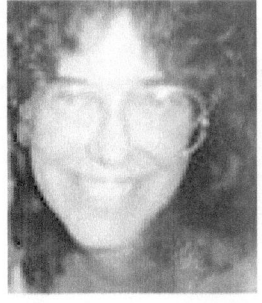

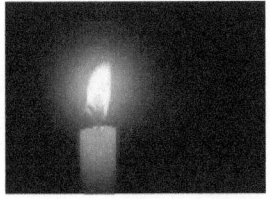

Pat Wagner, USA (1950 -2018), treated on Apitherapy for free over 20,000 patients suffering multiple sclerosis and other disorders.

They made an outstanding difference to mankind in modern times by researching, practicing, teaching, and promoting Apitherapy with altruism, future vision, bravery and passion against all odds, and against academic prejudices by contemporary peers. They were the new *Quixotes* and *Sanchoes* of Healing Arts, and they are paradigms for next generations of apitherapists. Modern Apitherapy owes them a great deal.

NOTES

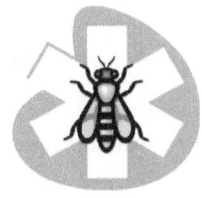

1. ADVENTURE IN APITHERAPY REALMS

Duermo en mi cama de roca
Mi sueño dulce y profundo:
Roza una abeja mi boca
Y crece en mi cuerpo el mundo

[Sleeping in my rock bed
My deep, sweet sleep
A bee my mouth scuffs
And world in my body swells]

José Martí (*Versos sencillos*, 1891)

DID YOU KNOW THAT?

- The median lethal dose (LD50) of bee venom or apitoxin for an adult human is 2.8 mg of venom per kg of body weight, i.e. a person weighing 60 kg has a 50 % chance of surviving injections totaling 168 mg of bee venom or some 600 bee stings. Only < 2 % of the world population (some studies show 0.7 %) is allergic to bee stings.
- Bees are the only invertebrates who understand the concept of zero: they recognize "no shapes" as a smaller value than "some shapes".

- Bee venom peptides as melittin and phospholipase A2 induce apoptosis in rheumatoid synovia cells, and in proliferative cells of breast, kidney, leukemia, liver, lung, prostate, and other cancers.
- Bee larvae develop into workers, in part, because their diet of pollen and honey, called bee bread, is rich in plant regulatory molecules called micro-RNAs, which delay development and keep their ovaries inactive. While the workers primarily consume bee bread, the queens feast on royal jelly secreted by the glands of nurse bees.
- Bee venom is an effective adjuvant treatment for Parkinson's disease, multiple sclerosis, Lyme disease, cancer, Lou-Gehrig's disease, attenuates neuroinflammation, inhibits apoptosis of dopaminergic neurons, restores normal dopamine levels, and protects against glutamate-induced neurotoxicity. Honey bees are the only bees or insects to die after stinging.
- Beekeepers have a lower risk of being diagnosed with arthritis, arthrosis, multiple sclerosis, asthma, goiter, psoriasis, cancer, HIV/AIDS, and other diseases than other persons.
- A bee weighs 80 mg and can transport 70 mg of nectar plus 20 mg of pollen in a flight, and would need 80 million visits to flowers to produce one kilogram of honey.
- The best wood in smokers for calming aggressive bees is carqueja (*Baccharis trimera*).
- Bees flap their two pairs of wings 11,400 times per minute and travel at 22 km per hour. A worker bee can reach a total of 800 km flown in her lifespan (4 - 5 months) and in total produces only half a teaspoon of honey.
- Drone sperm protects the queen bee from *Nosema apis* spores and other diseases.
- A company in Montana, USA, trains honey bees for detecting mine fields, explosives, and biological and chemical weapons with an over 97 % precision. The results show that bees are conditioned with TNT (trinitrotoluene), RDX (cyclotrimethylenetrinitramine, also known as T4, cyclonite or hexogen), DNT (dinitrotoluene), 2,4-DNT, 2,6-DNT, 4-amino-DNT, and other compounds soaked in syrup for allowing bees to detect environmental vapors from the chemical agent, explosive, or biological agent. Another laboratory, in New

Mexico, USA, uses bees for detecting TNT, C4, TATP, and other explosives and detonants.

- The olfactory sense of a bee is 10 times better than humans and three or four times better than a dog's.
- Honey sweetens 25 times more than refined sugar.
- Japanese honey bees defend against hornets by massively vibrating to elevate hive temperature to 47 degrees Celsius, lethal for hornets. Honey bees tolerate a higher temperature of 47.8 degrees Celsius and don't need a massive "kamikaze" attack on the hornets.
- Nanoparticles carrying melittin fuse with human immunodeficiency virus and destroy its protective envelope.
- Bumble bees (*Bombus* sp.) are better than computers at solving the Traveling Salesman Problem, a non-deterministic polynomial-time hard/complete algorithm. As bees visit flowers to collect nectar and pollen, they discover other flowers on route in the wrong order. It is unknown how they manage to quickly learn and fly the optimally shortest path between the 1000 flowers each bee visits during a flight, i.e. 40 flowers per minute.
- Bees distinguish blue, yellow, and white colors, they are blind to red and confuse green with yellow and blue.

IN THE BEGINNING

It is never too late for learning, and for ending ignorance. Even after my adolescence, I barely knew that honey bees and wasps were completely different insects, and who knows why, perhaps from TV cartoons, I believed that a bee had the stinger on her head, like a unicorn. I don't remember when I observed the interior of a hive or had a bee between my fingers, but it was much later that fate placed me in the path of Apitherapy.

My childhood memories of bees consisted of a few bees flying within Havana bakeries –empty, boring places during the many decades of Castroite regime, where bees were seldom attracted; these marvelous creatures were my non-acquaintances for many years. On the other hand, no one in my extended family or ancestors was a beekeeper or even a farmer: none from my paternal grandparents, Sephardic immigrants from Turkey (grandpa Moisés was a retail businessman and Esther was an oriental rug weaver), or from my maternal grandparents (Alfonso was a Spanish immigrant with trade as a dental technician and Romualda was a Cuban hospital attendant), plus a large extended family on both sides including a Spanish great-aunt who was an orphanage nun until her death. None had anything to do with bees or farms.

While working at the National Cadres Division of Cuba Ministry of Agriculture (known until 1975 as the National Institute for Land Reform), at a beautiful garden mansion expropriated in the Biltmore neighborhood in western Havana, for the first time I saw a hive, kept as an oddity close to the garden's swimming pool by the National Beekeeping Division's staff. But in those years my interests were "only" information science, hypnosis, parapsychology, and playwright, while I was enrolled in the University of Havana's BSc in Information/Library Science, which was a way to have access to information, a scarce resource in closed societies.

A couple of years later, I was working in another division of the Ministry of Agriculture (the Center for Agricultural Information and Documentation), as an information analyst at a little think-tank and writing digests from foreign scientific literature, article reviews, and even books. At that time, no specialist was processing the literature on beekeeping and, why not, I thought and took the opportunity of analyzing, digesting, and processing tens of journals on apiculture subscribed from all over the world.

Very interesting articles on Apitherapy did pop up before my eyes in journals *American Bee Journal, Pchelovodstvo, Apiacta, L'Abeille de France et l'Apiculteur, Journal of Apicultural Research, Gleanings in Bee Culture, Apicultura în România, Bee World, Apidologie, Apicultural Abstracts*, etc. Research replaced my initial curiosity. I was astounded to find out that Apitherapy was deceitfully ignored in Cuba and that propolis, bee bread, and other bee products, except exportable honey and beeswax, were discarded. My contacts with beekeeping officials corroborated that propolis had no value to them, which inspired the notion that a book on this bee product could be useful. For months I was searching, translating, and processing a huge volume of information including quality standards for propolis, and the result was my poorly designed and first book on Apitherapy, *Propóleo, un valioso producto apícola* (1979). Later, I met and befriended veteran beekeepers César Abreu and Pedro Redondo, who empirically knew a lot about the therapeutic properties of some bee products, but nobody had listened to them.

For years, the book went unnoticed in Cuba, and once again the paraphrased biblical quote came to reality, "No prophet is welcome in his home town": The International Bee Research Association (IBRA) purchased several dozens of copies and recommended the book among the top 24 books that developing countries should include in any basic library on beekeeping (*IBRA. Source Materials for Apiculture*, No. 8, 1981). Several years later, Frank Vernon wrote a very favorable book review ("...By far, the most complete review of propolis so far published", *Bee Talk* 65:2-3, March 1987).

An international war had indirect consequences and, consequently, Apitherapy became a welcome and opportune discipline in Cuba. Russians, the Soviet Union's Red Army, had occupied Afghanistan to impose its pro-Communist government, but events took a turn for the worse and the Afghan mujahedeen fought a bloody war against the powerful Red Army, a devastating and long war that exhausted Soviet economy and morale which ultimately led to a dramatic reduction of subsidies and aid to Cuba.

In those years and subsequent decades, Cuban economy subsisted in a precarious condition, as it depended on Soviet supplies and subventions. Imports and budgets were drastically reduced, and the Soviet Union could not cope with both a lost war in Afghanistan and the arms race with the United States (remember those years of "Star Wars"?), therefore the subsidies to Cuba and Eastern Europe satellites dwindled.

Imports of veterinary medicines and feedstuffs were seriously affected. At that time, veterinary doctors took notice of *Propóleo, un valioso producto apícola*, and started using propolis to heal newborn calves, infected wounds and parasites in cattle and other mammals, poultry, fish, and pets. Medical physicians learned that their veterinary colleagues were using propolis and had established some little factories of propolis tincture and other products, and immediately began prescribing propolis, pollen, and other bee products (without the Ministry of Public Health's approval!) for dermatitis, hypercholesterolemia, wounds, burns, parasitosis, and other disorders. Pretty soon in many hospitals in all Cuban provinces there were laboratories where propolis tincture, shampoo, soap, ointment, eye drops, capsules, emulsion, and candies were produced.

An increasing demand for cheaper medications to replace imports fueled an interest in learning more about Apitherapy and other fields of Complementary and Alternative Medicine.

The Veterinary Medicine Institute of Matanzas, a province located 83 km from Havana, was the first government institution to create a laboratory in Cuba to produce tinctures and other recipes from propolis and honey for animal use, however the demand for human use was ever-increasing. This Institute sponsored the first scientific symposia on propolis in 1988 and 1989 in Varadero beach, which boosted exposure in other national and international seminars, books, newspaper articles and magazines, radio and TV programs, even cartoons: Cuban Apitherapy had been born. At the same time, other propolis laboratories at the University of Havana, Apicultural Research Center in Havana, and in Pinar del Río, Matanzas, Sancti Spíritus, Camagüey, Holguín, and several other provinces were established.

Propolis, pollen, honey, bee venom, and other bee products became as popular in medication cabinets of Cuban doctors and patients as aspirin and cough medicine. In the Western Hemisphere, Argentina, Brazil, Chile, Cuba, Mexico, United States, and Uruguay developed into the most advanced countries in the field of Apitherapy.

I remember one morning in my office when a forestry engineer, Santiago Fabré, visited me and shared his life story: he had been sent to Angola with many other Cubans to exploit the valuable lumber in that West-African country, and he contracted malaria. Days passed and his high fever didn't recede, doctors were very pessimist regarding his prognosis, until somebody read in my neglected book *Propóleo, un valioso producto apícola* that propolis was "useful" for treating malaria. Oral propolis was included in Fabré's diet and, to doctors' amazement, not only he survived but his remission was rapid and remarkable. Shortly afterwards, Fabré was back in Cuba and leading a normal life. Of course, he became an advocate of propolis therapy, a good friend of mine, and often shared with me his readings and insights.

Propolis, pollen, honey, bee venom, and other bee products became so popular in medicine repositories and apothecaries of Cuban doctors, I continued to write other books: *Los productos de la colmena* (1988), *Investigaciones cubanas sobre el propóleo* (1989), *Propóleo: el oro púrpura de las abejas* (1989, 1991, 2005), and others. *Apiterapia para todos* was published in Cuba in 1996 and in Mexico in 2001. *Apiterapia 101 para todos* was published in the United States in 2007 and re-edited a decade later.

Mexican beekeeper and apitherapist Trinidad Terrazas, as she wrote in her "Prologue to Mexican Edition" of *Apiterapia para todos*, was vacationing in Cuba in 1997 and purchased all remaining copies of *Apiterapia para todos* available in Varadero beach bookstores. Later, she tried to contact the author to purchase more copies of the book for her stores in Guadalajara and all her letters were returned from Cuba: I had left the country in 1993. To her surprise, I had never seen the published book, as Cuban government publishers had dishonored the contracts, and it was Mrs. Terrazas, "La Tía Trini", who sent me some copies of the book and her company prepared the Mexican edition of *Apiterapia para todos* in 2001.

In 1990, the Open International University for Complementary Medicines granted me a PhD Honoris Causa, and two years later a degree of MD/*Medicina Alternativa* plus a life membership in the organization Medicina Alternativa International. In those years, I was appointed a member in the board of the International Apitherapy Healthcare and Bee Acupuncture Association.

As living in Cuba meant global isolation and the financial inability to pay membership fees, in 1991 a dear colleague and pioneer of American Apitherapy, Charles Mraz (1905 - 1999), graciously welcomed me as a member of the American Apitherapy Society (AAS). After immigrating to the United States in 1993, I continued lecturing on Apitherapy in many countries, and in 2009 the AAS elected me to serve in its board for several years.

Letters and comments from readers are very rewarding, as well as meeting people who have learned Apitherapy from my books and healed themselves or relatives. While I was living in Cuba, Lucy Levy, a lady in charge of social programs for wounded guerrillas from El Salvador, asked me for several copies of *Propóleo, un valioso producto apícola*, as she knew that war wounds could be healed by putting into practice my texts. In the 2000's, people in the United States told the tale of two Cubans, not related each other, who arrived in Miami as rafters —a journey of two hundred kilometers crossing the Florida Straits in hand-made rustic rafts--, and who had brought my Apitherapy books well wrapped in plastic to protect them from the sea water amongst their scarce belongings. Recently, I met a beekeeper in Santo Domingo who had managed to purchase all my Apitherapy books and had memorized full chapters of some of them.

In late 2005 - 2016, three apitherapists from diverse countries and I founded Bees for Life – World Apitherapy Network (www.facebook. com / groups / BeesForLifeWorldApitherapy), a nonprofit educational and charitable organization which provides assistance in emergency situations by using Apitherapy. Members of this organization have been lecturing to large audiences in all continents, and have used Apitherapy to help populations in countries hit by disasters and poverty.

But the dream of Apitherapy having a place in public health has not been achieved, and much effort and actions will be needed in the years ahead.

Complementary and Alternative Medicine focuses on Homeopathy, Acupuncture, Akabane, Tibb, Macrobiotics, Iridology, Moratherapy, Kirlian Halography, Holistic Medicine, Psychic Healing, Ayurveda, Cryotherapy, Green Medicine, Qi-gong, Chromotherapy, Quantic Healing, Bioenergetics Medicine, Unami, Magnetotherapy, Siddhah, Tai-chi-chuan, Chiropractics, Shiatsu, Meditation, Kiodoraku, and others. Seldom is Apitherapy mentioned.

Apitherapy is a young discipline —less than a hundred years since Bodog Beck, MD, suggested this term for the bee venom therapy and for the therapy with other bee products. Nevertheless, 6000 years ago, the Chinese recommended honey as a medication, and Egyptian, Hittite, Hebrew, Greek, Hindu, Persian, Roman, and other civilizations had considered the properties of honey, beeswax, propolis, beeswax, even ground bees.

Many peoples have practiced a veneration to bees: Melissa, goddess of bees in Greek mythology, fed Jupiter with honey, and Aristaeus was the god of beekeeping; Mellona or Mellonia was the Roman goddess of bees; Ah-Muzen-Cab and Colel Cab, Mayan god and goddess of bees; Zosima of Solovki, an Ukrainian saint; Nantosuelta, a Roman-German bee goddess; Bubilas and Austeja, bee god and goddess of ancient Polish, Latvians, Lithuanians, and Silesians; Vishnu was a deity in India; Bhramari, Hindu goddess of bees, as these invertebrates were a totem for Brahmins and Juangs of India, Zambian Ba-Kaondas, and Suks, Nandis and other tribes in Africa.

Apitherapy deserves a serious evaluation by all scientific and medical communities, as it has much to offer for the healing of hundreds of disorders at a low cost, high effectiveness, and reduced side-effects. Let's do it before Big Pharma and Big Medical Protocol Guild take control as a greedy industry. This book is a complement to all other Apitherapy's authors and provides clinical forms, progress notes, medical evaluations, allergy tables, SOAP notes, Apipuncture diagrams, measure conversion tables, and other useful tools for the field Apitherapy practitioner. *Apitherapy 101* series is for outreach, introduction, and thus I have omitted bibliographic references and sources in benefit of a more comfortable reading, 30 % illustrated.

After this Introduction, my only advice is: go, explore and study everywhere, learn from everyone, teach everybody, share with all, and practice more and more on humbleness and altruism, as every day there will be an amazing new information.

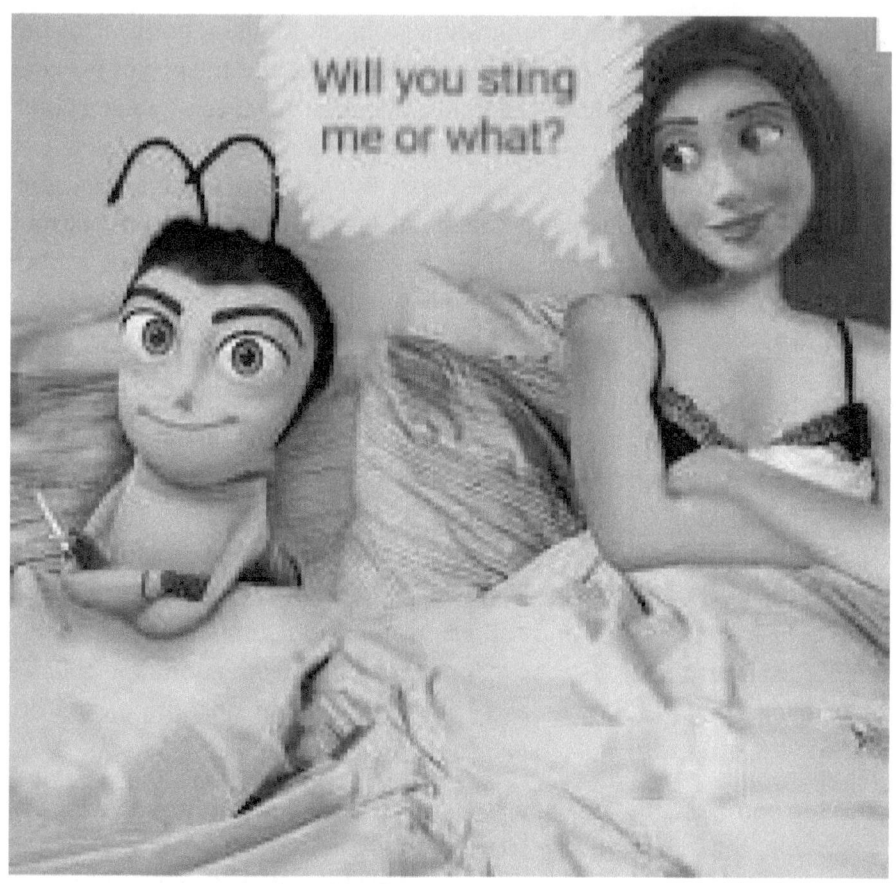

A BEE CAN HEAL A WHOLE COMMUNITY.

- Una colmena puede curar a toda una comunidad.
- דבורה יכולה לרפא קהילה שלמה
- Une abeille peut guérir toute une communauté.
- Eine Honigbiene kann eine ganze Gemeinschaft heilen.
- 蜜蜂可以治愈整個社區。
- Může léčit celou komunitu.
- Un api può guarire un'intera comunità.
- ผึ้งสามารถรักษาทั้งชุมชนได้
- Pszczoła miodna może uzdrawiać całą społeczność.
- Albină poate vindeca o întreagă comunitate.
- Včely môžu liečiť celé spoločenstvo.
- ንብ፞ አንድ ማህበረሰብን መፈወስ ይችላሉ.
- Meda može izliječiti cijelu zajednicu.
- Unha abella pode curar toda unha comunidade.
- 蜜蜂可以治愈整个社区。
- Una abella pot curar tota una comunitat.
- ن ل العسل يمكن أن يشفي المجتمع بأكمله.
- En honungsbinnkaka kan läka en hel gemenskap.
- Gall gwenynen fwyn wella cymuned gyfan.
- ຮ່ງເຜິ້ງສາມາດປິ່ນປົວຊຸມຊົນທັງໝົດໄດ້.
- Naħal tal-għasel jista 'jfejjaq komunità sħiħa.
- Abaraska batek komunitate oso bat sendatu dezake.
- Улей пчел может излечить целую общину.
- Një zgjua bletësh mund të shërojë një komunitet të tërë.
- Μια κυψέλη μέλισσας μπορεί να θεραπεύσει μια ολόκληρη κοινότητα.
- Pesä voi parantaa koko yhteisön.
- Býflugur getur læknað heil samfélag.
- کندو زنبور عسل می تواند یک کل جامعه را درمان کند.
- Един пчелен кошер може да излекува цяла общност.
- Sarang lebah madu bisa menyembuhkan seluruh komunitas.
- شاتو شاتو کولی شي ټوله ټولنه روغ کړي.
- En honningbikeklub kan helbrede et helt fællesskab.
- Зөгийн бал зөгий нь бүхэл бүтэн нийгэмийг эдгээж чадна.
- I-isidleke singaphulukisa umphakathi wonke.
- Вулик медоносець може зцілити цілу громаду.
- A mézelő méhcsaládok gyógyíthatják az egész közösséget.
- Abelo povas resanigi tutan komunumon.

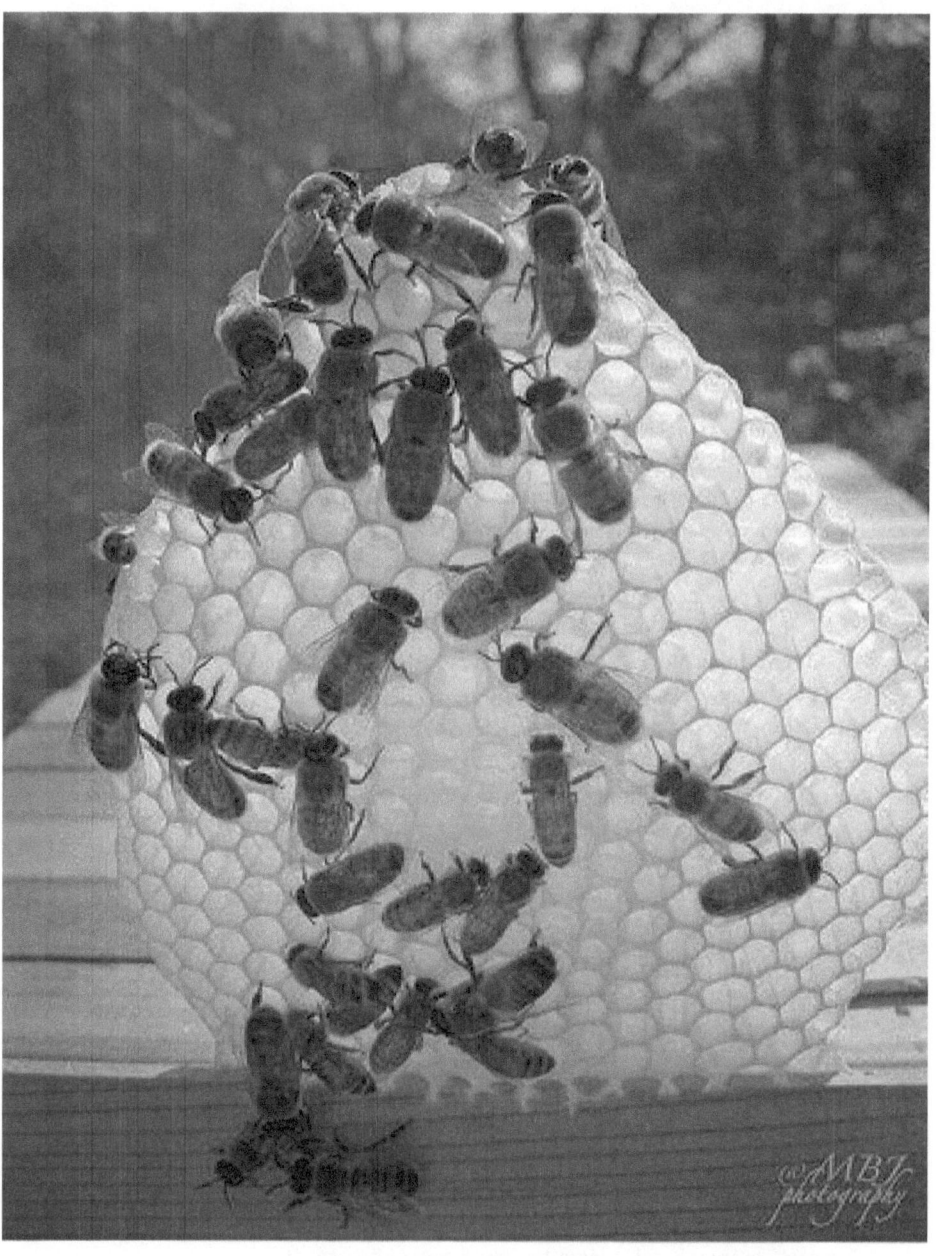

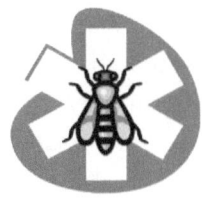

2. APITHERAPY

Apitherapy is the Complementary and Alternative Medicine that promotes the use of bee products (honey, honeydew honey, stingless bee honey, mead, propolis, géopropolis, hive air, beeswax, *zabrus* or honeycomb capping, pollen, bee bread, apitoxin or bee venom, drone larvae, royal jelly, and whole bees) for nutrition, enhancement of health and life quality, prevention and treatment of diseases, and is also used for cosmetic treatments. Apitherapy comprises, among its many techniques, the apitoxitherapy or bee venom therapy, and the apipuncture or acupuncture by bee stings, micro-stings and apitoxin microinjections, massage with honey, propolis oil and apitoxin oil, use of stipers, inhalation, topical applications, suppositories, oral ingestion, injections, capsules, drops, and as a synergetic coadjutant of food and prescription drugs.

Clinical forms in this book include informed consents for Apitherapy, notes, progress notes, health history, prescriptions currently taken, evaluation, SOAP (subjective, objective, assessment, and plan) forms, maintenance logs, acupuncture diagrams for use in Apitherapy, and other documents and reference tables.

Apitherapy practitioners can use all these 60+ forms directly from this book or to make copies for use with patients.

There are many good books and article reviews on Apitherapy in different languages. For further information and updates, many sources are available: Apitherapy News (www.apitherapynews .com), PubMed-NCBI (www.ncbi.nlm.nih.gov / m / pubmed), websites of national Apitherapy societies (see Chapter 12), National Honey Board (www.nhb.org), International Bee Research Association (www. ibra.org.uk), Apimondia Standing Commission of Apitherapy (www.apimondia.com/en/activities/ scientific-commissions/apitherapy); Thomson Reuters Clarivate (www.clarivate.com), Web of Science (www.WebofScience .com), WorldCat (www.worldcat.org), www.Science.gov, MedlinePlus (www.medlineplus.gov), Archive of Healing, Ritual, and Transformation (www.ahrt.ucla.edu), Google Scholar (www.scholar.google.com), Kosmet (www.kosmet.com), Natural Medical Protocols (www.naturalopinion.com), Espacenet (www.worldwide.espacenet.net), Scopus Elsevier (www.scopus.com), TCM Database System (www.cintcmac.cn), National Institutes of Health (NIH) Clinical Research Trials and You (www.nih.gov/health/clinicaltrials), Facebook.com / apitherapy101, Facebook.com / groups / BeesForLifeWorld-Api- therapy, and Facebook.com / The-Open-International-University -for-Complementary-Medicines.

Of course, there are many other valuable databases on Apitherapy research and bee products in English and other languages, for example Sudoc (www.sudoc.abes.fr), Russian Science Citation Index (Российский индекс научного цитирования: www.elibrary.ru) and VINITI Database RAS (www2.viniti.ru), SciELO (www.scielo.org) and Biotechgate Global Database (www.germanbiotech.com/de), and other hundreds of links.

All bee products are synergistic to medical drugs and procedures; and Apitherapy integrates many practices from allopathic or Western medicine, Ayurveda, traditional Chinese, Korean, African, Iranian, indigenous, and Siddha medicines, and other complementary and alternative medicines.

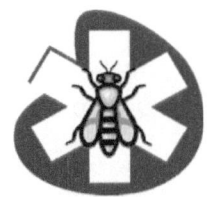

3. BEEHIVE PRODUCTS

There are at least 15 beehive products used in Apitherapy: **apitoxin** (bee venom, and from it Bee Venom Therapy as defined by Bodog Beck), **bee pollen** and **bee bread**, **propolis** and **géopropolis**, **royal jelly**, *Apis mellifera* **honey** and **stingless bee honey**, **honeydew honey**, **mead**, **beeswax**, **honeycomb capping**, **drone larvae** (also called **Apilarnil**), **hive air**, and **whole bees**. Honey bees have been in existence for over 100 million years, and it appears that they paved the path for men and animals on this planet to have a healthy existence.

In fact, a hive has all the nutrients needed for living beings including us: bee pollen, the best source of essential amino acids (proteins), vitamins, enzymes, minerals, and other nutrients; honey is a unique complex of carbohydrates, vitamins, minerals, and many other compounds. Propolis is the best antibiotic and wound healer ever known; and royal jelly, beeswax, drone larvae, and the other products meet human needs better than the best gourmet buffet restaurant and medicine cabinet. Regarding our health, it is possible to heal a community from a hive: from wounds, diabetes and cancer to arthritis, infectious diseases and immune disorders, for only mentioning some of the hundreds of disorders treatable with bee products.

One of my favorite public presentations is how to treat emergencies, injuries from disasters, wars, famines, natural catastrophes, by using only a hive as a first-aid cabinet. See the last two pages of this book for a glance on this.

All books, article reviews, and websites on Apitherapy have similar information on the composition, biological properties and therapeutic uses of these 15 products, and it is positive to replicate such an information once and again. In Apitherapy textbooks, online sources, presentations, videos, courses, and throughout national

Apitherapy societies and international networks of apitherapists, detailed information on these products and their collection, conservation, processing, composition, properties, use, and contraindications is available.

3.1 APITOXIN OR BEE VENOM

Apitoxin enzymes are 30 times more active than snake venom and stronger than any antibiotic. Honey bees sting only in self-defense of their hive and die when their guts are disemboweled in attempting to pull out their serrate stingers stuck deep in human or animal skin. Nonetheless, there are methods for extracting bee venom and protecting their stingers without any harm to worker bees.

Dufour and venom glands, and stinger intervene in the self-defense of honey bee colonies by providing workers and queens with a powerful weapon. Apitoxin or bee venom is produced in the venom sac of workers and queens and it contains at least 18 pharmacologically active components, including various enzymes, peptides and amines, but in total there are more than 60 identifiable components in bee venom.

The main component of bee venom responsible for pain is melittin and it accounts for 52 % of venom peptides; it induces the production of cortisone in the stung organism, has cytotoxic effect and induces apoptosis of cancer cells, has an antimicrobial effect, and it is a strong anti-inflammatory agent, 100 times more potent than hydrocortisol.

Phospholipase A2 comprises 10 - 12 % of peptides and it is the most destructive component of apitoxin. It degrades the phospholipids, breaks down the membranes of blood cells, resulting in cell destruction, causes decreased blood pressure, inhibits blood coagulation, activates arachidonic acid which is metabolized in the cyclooxygenase-cycle to form prostaglandins, which regulate the body's inflammatory response. Additionally, unlike most larger molecules in the venom, it causes the release of pain-inducing agents.

Hyaluronidase aids the action of the venom by catalyzing the breakdown of protein-polysaccharide complexes in tissue, allowing the venom to penetrate further into the flesh.

Apamin, a mild neurotoxin, has antiatherosclerotic effect, inhibits complement C_3 activity, increases cortisol production in the adrenal gland and blocks calcium-dependent potassium channels, thus enhancing synaptic transmission. Adolapin acts as an anti-inflammatory agent and analgesic because it blocks cyclooxygenase.

Substances, such as hyaluronidase, phospholipase A2, histamine, peptide 401 or mast cell degranulating protein, and other compounds are involved in the inflammatory response of venom, with the softening of tissue and the facilitation of flow of the other substances. Mast cell degranulating can also cause mast cells in the body to release more histamine, worsening inflammation.

Histamine and other biogenic amines released by the body during the allergic response, can cause itchiness, pain, and inflammation. The proteins in the sting can cause an allergic reaction, leading to the release of even more histamine, and possible anaphylaxis. Secapin has antimicrobial effect and inhibits serine protease.

Finally, there are measurable amounts of the neurotransmitters dopamine, norepinephrine and serotonin.

Apitoxin activates the immune system, stimulates the pituitary-cortical system and secretion of cortisol, has an immediate inflammatory effect and secondary anti-inflammatory effect, decreases pain intensity, and improves blood circulation.

Bee venom therapy is effective for the treatment of arthritis, multiple sclerosis, premenstrual syndrome, epilepsy, chronic pain, migraine, high blood cholesterol, rhinosinusitis, atherosclerosis, polyneuritis, Ménière syndrome, radiculitis, infectious spondylitis, neuralgia, endarteritis, polyarthritis, Alzheimer and some other dementias, malaria, Lyme disease, intercostal myalgia, myositis, HIV/AIDS, Parkinson disease, topical ulcers, slowly healing wounds, thrombophlebitis, keratoconjunctivitis, iritis, iridocyclitis, asthma, bursitis, ligament injuries, mastitis, some types of cancer, Friedrich and Strümpel ataxias, sore throat, immunodepression, high blood viscosity and coagulability, narrowed capillaries and arteries, among many other disorders.

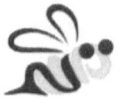

3.2 BEE BREAD

Bee bread is for pollen like yogurt, Smetana and kefir are for milk. "Bee's Smetana", it sounds good and it is much better than Smetana. However, the difference between bee bread and pollen is greater than the difference between bee pollen and flower pollen. Bee bread is a fermented mixture of plant pollen, honey, and bee saliva, but it is superior to bee pollen and honey thanks to pollen fermentative hydrolysis and acid hydrolysis, triple nutritive value and greater antibiotic properties than bee pollen.

A bee transports 8 to 15 mg of fresh pollen in each leg. Bee bread cells are filled with the pollen of nine bees, mixed with honey, and with 9-oxo-2-decenoic and 10-hydroxy-2-decenoic acids from a bee's salivary glands. This pollen is transformed by 33 - 35 degrees Celsius temperature, high humidity, monosaccharides convert into lactic acid, vitamin K content increases, and within 12 hours lacto bacteria, yeasts, airborne bacteria appear, then lacto acid bacteria (*Streptococci* sp.) develop, acidity and vitamin B increase. Finally, streptococci disappear and lactobacilli develop, but between days 7 and 15 lactobacteria disappear and acidity reaches a pH 4 - 4.3, lactic acid is increases to a 3.2 % and bee bread keeps its antibiotic properties and keeps its freshness in a fresh dry place carbohydrates, plus lipids, minerals, vitamins, it is rich in B-complex vitamins, essential amino acids, and fatty acids, high provitamin A, vitamins E and C; 43 - 70 % fructose, glucose, galactose, sucrose, maltose, raffinose, inosine, and other sugars; high lactic acid (0.7 - 1.1 %), and an increased stability due to fermentative hydrolysis of polysaccharides altogether with an acid hydrolysis.

Bee bread is rich in quercetin myricetin, kaempferol, isorhamnetin, herbacetin glycoside derivatives and other flavonol derivatives, and has triple nutritional and antibiotic properties than pollen; it has the same biological properties as pollen, increases immune properties, reduces fatigue and it's very valuable for treating colitis, chronic constipation, diarrheas, hepatitis, nervous disorders, anemia, breast adeno- carcinoma, non-small lung cancer, hepatocellular carcinoma, cervical carcinoma, and other disorders.

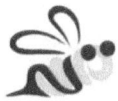

3.3 BEESWAX

B eeswax is a secretion of wax glands of young worker bees: small wax flakes are released from abdominal rings, while other bees collect and chew them with some pollen and propolis for using beeswax in constructing those perfect hexahedral cells in combs.

It contains some 300 compounds including 71 % linear wax monoesters, hydroxy monoesters deriving from palmitic, 15-hydroxypalmitic, and oleic acids, and complex wax esters containing 15-hydroxypalmitic acid and diols, diesters and triesters, 14 % of free waxy acids, plus lactones, cholesteryl esters, colorants, free alcohols, minerals, and other compounds. It Is very rich in vitamin A (600 % more than beef), and contains more than eleven proteins and 50 aroma components. Chemical composition also includes 14 % hydrocarbons (heptacosane, nonacosane, hentriacontane, pentacosane and tricosane).

For thousands of years, ancient civilizations in India, Egypt, China, Greece, Rome, and other American and European cultures, have used ear wax cone-candling. It is used for removing excess cerumen, alleviating tinnitus, and viral, bacterial, fungal/yeast infections in ears. In those cultures, beeswax has been also known as a major remedy in ointments for inflammation, joint pain, bruises, burns, and cracked heels. Ancient Egyptians and Persians used it for embalming and mummifying corpses, and Romans for modelling death masks and as writing tablets.

In addition to its use in cosmetics, dentistry, furniture, welding, electronics, optics, radiotechnology, rail transportation, textile industry, perfumes, aviation, leather tanning, food industry, it has therapeutic uses.

It has antimicrobial properties and inhibitory effects against *Aspergillus niger*, *Candida albicans*, *Salmonella enterica*, *Staphylococcus aureus*, and other bacteria and fungi, and preservative effects.

Chewing or inhaling a mix of beeswax and honey is good for sinusitis, asthma, hay fever, and nasopharyngeal affections. It promotes saliva secretion, increased stomach activity and metabolism, betters blood circulation, muscle working capacity, removes tooth tartar, strengthens the gums, and helps quitting smoking addiction. But beeswax has many other therapeutic applications as shown in Apitherapy textbooks.

3.4. DRONE LARVAE OR APILARNIL

For thousands of years bee drone larvae have been a beekeeper's Viagra (sildenafil citrate) and Cialis (tadalafil). In a bee colony, a thousand drones live between 28 and 62 days and their main function is competing with all other drones to be among the fastest twenty who can reach and copulate the queen during the nuptial flight. However, they perform other tasks in the hive such as producing heat, warming the brood, and distributing nectar to workers. Furthermore, they eat much pollen, honey, and royal jelly, and are more expensive to a bee colony than kings and princes for modern queen-led monarchies in human society.

After this event, drones are sacrificed by workers or starved to death outside their hive. They are unable to collect nectar and pollen and have no sting to defend themselves.

Drone larvae are rich in amino acids, carbohydrates, lipids, minerals, and vitamins. Their composition includes 17 essential amino acids and their nutritive peak is reached 10 days after drone eggs are laid.

Since the 1980s, many products use drone larvae after Nicolae V. Ilieşiu lyophilized drone larvae and patented Apilarnil. Ilieşiu had observed that his neighbor's ducks, fed mainly on drone larvae, had a faster development, and he thought of studying and processing those larvae for use in human nutrition and health.

The main biological properties of drone larvae are: strong antiviral, psycho-stimulating and bio-stimulating activity, increased immune system and resistance to diseases, increased libido, spermatogenesis, erection, time of copulation, suprarenal glands, hypophysis and anabolism, regulate the menstrual cycle in women, impact on memory and nervous system, increased appetite, energy, and muscle weight gain.

Drone larvae or Apilarnil are rich in proteins, carbohydrates, lipids, vitamins, and minerals. They contain vitamins such as vitamin A (5400 IU/g), vitamin B1 (2.0 mg/kg), vitamin B2 (9.0 mg/kg), provitamin A or ß-carotene (4.0 mg/kg), and choline (1790 mg/kg); minerals such as cadmium, calcium, copper, phosphorus, iron, magnesium, potassium, sodium, and zinc. Their amino acid composition and biological properties are comparable to royal jelly.

Drone larvae are used for treating many disorders including neurosis (all types), sexual asthenia, erectile dysfunction, low spermatogonia, sterility, skin affections, premenstrual syndrome, climacteric syndrome, physical weakness and asthenia, anorexia, digestive dysfunctions, cholecystitis, migraine, premature aging, arteriosclerosis, memory decline, endarteritis, arterial hypertension and hypotension, hepatitis, vision and hearing diminution, osteochondritis, hypoproteinemia, diabetes, obesity, gout, flu and other viral infections, immune disorders, bacterial and fungal glosostomatitis, chronic pharyngitis, rhinitis, sinusitis, laryngitis, allergic hyper sensibility reactions, and malnutrition.

Contraindications include iron-deficiency, corticosuprarenal hyperfunction, cerebrovascular hypertension, cardiac insufficiency, and renal insufficiency. Adult daily doses are 300 to 800 mg.

3.5 GÉOPROPOLIS

Nests of stingless bees consist of a mix of propolis and beeswax, as bees store that géopropolis in large deposits forming their nests. Géopropolis is produced by stingless bees from the resinous material of plants, adding soil or clay. Stingless bees construct horizontal combs made of cerumen or geopropolis for their nests, and honey pots instead of honeycombs for storing honey.

Géopropolis has properties very like propolis and beeswax, it is rich in mono-terpenes and sesquiterpenes, phenolic compounds, triterpenes, saponins,5,7-dihydroxy-6(3-methyl-2-butenyl)-8-(4-cinnamoyl-3-meth- yl-1-oxobutyl)-4-propyl-coumarin, 5,7-dihydroxy-6-(4-cinnamoyl-3-me- thyl1-oxobutyl)-4-phenylcoumarin, mammeigin, hydroxymammeigin, mammeisin, cinnamoyloxymammeisin, mammein, prenylated benzo- phenone ent-nemorosone, and other compounds found and others not found in propolis.

Biological activity of géopropolis includes anti-antibacterial (against *Streptococcus mutans*), anti-inflammatory, antinociceptive, and antitumor (by inducing apoptosis and cell cycle arrest of human glioblastoma, bone tumors, colon cancer, venereal transmissible tumors, laryngeal epidermoid carcinoma, and other types of cancer). The presence of benzophenones is associated with the antiproliferative (anti-cancer) activity of géopropolis.

3.6 HIVE AIR

Although the use of hive air has extended and become popular in many countries, first time I read about it was from "Tiroler Bienenwelt", a spa in Söll, Austria, offering its clients "bee air" (*Bienenluft* in German), a treatment of one hour per session, twice a day for two weeks, and consisting of an aerosol connected directly to a hive and extracting from it all volatile compounds of bee pheromones, honey, royal jelly, propolis, pollen, bee bread, bee venom, and other bee products. Honey has over 500 volatile compounds depending on bee species and nectar sources. These compounds include cis-linalool oxide, 2-phenylacetaldehyde, trans-linalool oxide, hotrienol, and furan-2,5-dicarbaldehyde.

Apitoxin or bee venom contains many volatile compounds and volatile alarm pheromones (4 – 8 %), such as isopentyl acetate, 2-nonanol, and n-butyl acetate, which trigger defensive responses from nearby insects.

In propolis, 10 % of compounds are volatile oils, and sesquiterpenes predominate in the volatile oils, followed by aromatic compounds, such as benzyl acetate, benzyl benzoate and benzyl alcohol, monoterpenes, monoterpenoids, phenols, long-chain alkanes, oxygenated mono- terpenes, terpenoids, oxygenated aliphatic hydrocarbons, long chain hydrocarbons, oxygenated hydrocarbons, oxygenated aromatic alcohols and esters. Their aroma and significant biological activity of propolis volatile compounds make them important for this resin characterization.

Volatile compounds are inhaled by using a simple device connected to the top cover of hives which pumps the hive air thanks to a little motor (from an old vacuum cleaner, inverted fan, or a CPAP (continuous positive airway pressure machine) and taking the air to the patient's face mask, as shown in the pictures.

Hive air is useful mainly for respiratory tract disorders and its properties are antimicrobial, antioxidant, antifungal, anxiolytic, anti-inflammatory, and many others.

3.7 HONEY

You could replicate a well-known 1971 Bulgarian experiment: place pieces of fish, kidney, liver, and other animal tissues in a container with honey, and the same kind of animal tissues in control group will be in a container with "artificial honey" (a mix of sugars such as glucose, laevulose, all other sugars composing honey, plus saline solution). In the experiment, the pieces covered with honey kept their freshness at room temperature for four years, and the pieces in the control group covered with "artificial honey" started decomposition on the fifth or eighth day.

In Egyptian pharaoh Tutankhamun's tomb, several honey chalices were found in 1922 and its honey was in good condition despite being 33 centuries old. A similar discovery was the honey in perfect conditions, after 2600 years, in amphoras in a Greek temple near to present-day Naples. When Alexander Magnum died in Babylon (323 BCE), he was transported in a gold sarcophagus filled with honey, then seized in Memphis and Alexandria, in Egypt, and later taken to Macedon. His body remained intact for this long period of time.

Honey's composition consists of flower nectar transformed in a supersaturated solution of fructose and glucose (only less than 20 % water) through repeated digestion and regurgitation by worker bees. This supersaturated solution contains also other sugars like sucrose, maltose, trehalose, N-acetylneuraminic acid, xylose, N-acetyl-galactosamine, N-acetylglucosamine, nigerose, oriose, turanose, panose, levocestose, and many others, enzymes like glucose oxidase, diastase (amylase), α-glucosidase, catalase, and acid phosphatase, invertase, amino acids and peptides like proline, glutamic acid, alanine, phenylalanine, tyrosine, leucine, isoleucine, defensin-1 and royal jelly protein isoforms. Also, some vitamins: B1, B2, PP or B3, B5, B6, C, K, folic acid, biotin; and minerals Ag, Al, Au, Be, Bi, Bo, Ca, Cl, Co, Cr, Cu, Fe, Ga, Ge, I, K, Li, Md, Mg, Mn, Na, Ni, Os, P, Pa, Pb, S, Si, Sr, St, Ti, V, Zn, Zr, and others.

Many beekeepers, apitherapists, and other people are familiar with all this information, but my guess is that only few persons, including medical doctors, know that honey is good for diabetic patients, within caloric allowances, and reduces blood glucose in patients with diabetes: fructose is a potential anti-diabetic agent, and the synergy of fructose/glucose balance promotes liver glucose metabolism. As honey has prebiotic properties and contains oligosaccharides, it has been hypothesized that its fructo-oligosaccharides, galacto-oligosaccharides, and lactulose have a preventive role against diabetes mellitus, insulin resistance, and obesity, by acting as prebiotics on the intestinal flora. These compounds could be linked to honey antidiabetic, antihyperlipidemic and hepatoprotective virtues.

In addition to its being high in energy carbohydrates (3.3 cal/g), rich in sugars, natural acids, minerals, proteins, enzymes, amino acids, and other substances, honey incorporates into the blood stream within 15 minutes. Refined sugars take two to four hours to be metabolized for converting sucrose into more digestible forms of glucosides and then assimilate them, with a great effort by pancreatic islets (known as islets of Langerhans), and this effort can exhaust the pancreatic islets and originate arthritis, diabetes mellitus, obesity, heart attacks, cancer, etc.

Tupelo (*Nyssa aquatica*) honey never crystallizes thanks to its high fructose content (44 %), it is recommended for diabetics, and it has an exquisite taste and other excellent organoleptic properties.

Some honeys have a very remarkable bactericidal activity: honeys of manuka (*Leptospermum scoparium*), red mangrove (*Rhizophora mangle*), tualang (*Koompassia excelsa*), kanuka (*Kunzea ericoides*), walnut (*Juglans regia*), pine (*Pinus* sp.), avocado (*Persea americana*), heather (*Calluna vulgaris*), akurai (*Psoralea melliferous drupacea*), argan (*Argania spinosa*), aroeira (*Schinus terebinthifolius*), eucalyptus (*Eucalyptus* sp.), mango (*Mangifera indica*), ulmo (*Eucryphia cordifolia*), buckwheat (*Fagopyrum* sp.), hawthorn (*Crataegus* sp.), kamahi (*Weinmannia racemosa*), kapok (*Ceiba pentandra*), clover *Trifolium* spp.), alfalfa (*Medicago sativa*), thyme (*Thymus vulgaris*), almond (*Amygdalus communis*), musk thistle (*Carduus nutans*), ironwood (*Olney* tesota), pohutukawa (*Metrosideros excelsa*), rata (*Metrosideros umbellata*), romerillo (*Bidens pilosa*), rubber (*Hevea* brasiliensis), sassafras (*Sassafras albidum*), Christ's thorn jujube (*Ziziphus spina-christi*), sourwood (*Oxydendrum arboreum*), tamarisk (*Tamarix* ramo-sissima), white birch (Betula pubescente), oak (Quercus lobate), strawberry (Fragaria ananassa), tupelo (Nyssa sp.), cedar of Lebanon (Cedrus libani), and acacia (Acacia spp.). Furthermore, all honeys have antimicrobial, antifungal and antiviral activity, wound healing, apoptosis of cancer cells, burn healing, cicatrizing, and other properties.

The antimicrobial activity of honey is provided by hydrogen peroxide, hypopharyngeal gland defensin-1, trihydroxyketone, methylglyoxal, acetic acid, 2,3-dihydro-3,5-dihydroxy-6-methyl-4H-pyran-4-one, 2-propanone, butanal, 1,3-benzenediamine, propanenitrile, 2-furan- methanol, propanoic acid, 1,3-butanediol, 1-(1-cyclopentenyl)-1-propanol, and 5-hydroxy- methylfurfural, and glycoproteins with high-mannose N-glycans. Thanks to these compounds, some honeys are very effective against methicillin-resistant Staphylococcus aureus (MRSA), Pseudomonas aeruginosa, Klebsiella pneumoniae, vancomycin-resistant enterococci, and extended-spectrum β-lactamase-producing Proteus mirabilis, and Escherichia coli.

Flavonoids in honey like apigenin, chrysin, galangin, kaempferol, and quercetin account for its antifungal action against pathogenic Candida albicans, C. parapsilosis, C. tropicalis, Rhodotorula sp., Aureobasidium pullulans, and Cladosporium cladosporioides.

Some honeys have antiprotozoal activity against the intestinal parasite Giardia lamblia and nematicide activity against Caenorhabditis elegans.

A very popular use of honey is for healing wounds and burns directly on the injury or by using medical-grade dressings. Manuka (Leptospermum scoparium) honey is exceptionally antibacterial potent, it is an antiseptic as potent as 10 % phenol and it is often used in commercial wound dressings. In infected wounds, it acts as an antioxidant hyperosmolar medium promoting healing and angiogenesis. Manuka, an endemic tree in New Zealand, is also known as New Zealand tea tree. Its honey is very active against a wide spectrum of bacteria and fungi, hence its use in treating bacterial diarrheas, rehydration of patients, prevention of dental cavities, and other applications. It is especially active against Staphylococcus aureus, Streptococcus pyogenes, and Helicobacter pylori; it can be used to treat ulcers, wound healing, eye infections, and diarrheas.

Another honey showing excellent properties is tualang (*Koompassia excelsa*) honey, a Malaysian tree reaching up 80 meters high and 200 cm in diameter, and its main property is stimulating and strengthening of immune system. Tualang tree is known under other names like bee tree, dëoh, ginoo, kayu, manggis, mengaris, menggeris, raja, sialang, tapang, and toale. The same can be stated of kanuka, also known as burgan or white tea tree (*Kunzea erycids*) honey, with a biological activity very like manuka and tualang honeys.

Honey is ideal to dress open wounds, abrasions, and puncture wounds, as it speeds wound healing and doesn't adhere to new tissue when the dressing is changed. Lesser scars are left in comparison with other treatments as it creates a very viscous barrier to prevent bacterial penetration and colonization in the wound's surface, and it increases local wound circulation. Honey reduces inflammation around wounds and drains lymphatic fluid and debris from the wound. In addition, it stimulates regeneration of damaged tissue, new capillary vessels, and collagen fibers and fibroblasts needed for forming new connective tissue.

Honey is used in surgeries since immemorial times. Very useful in surgery of vulva carcinoma, post-surgical treatment with honey prevents infections and acts as a germicide. It has extended use for diabetic ulcers, varicose legs, leprosy, sickle cell anemia, amputations, bedsore wounds, malignant ulcers, fistulas, surgical wounds, cuts, abrasions, puncture wounds, firearm wounds, traumatisms, and cracked nipples.

Phenolics are the most abundant phytochemicals (50 to 500 mg/kg) and very important contributors to the antioxidant capacity of honey. Honey has anticancer properties thanks to its content of trihydroxyketone, polyphenols caffeic acid and its phenyl esters, caffeoylquinic acid derivatives, rosmarinic acid and derivatives, ellagic acid, as well as the flavonoids chrysin, luteolin, acacetin, fisetin, myricetin, wogonin, apigenin, hesperidin, galangin, quercetin, kaempferol, pinobanksin, and pinocembrin.

The anti-inflammatory activity of honey is explained by the presence of apigenin, chrysin, daidzein, genistin, kaempferol, luteolin, quercetin, and other flavonoids, and glycopeptides, glycoproteins, peptides defensin-1, and apalbumin or royal jelly protein isoforms.

3.8 HONEYDEW HONEY

Also known as forest honey amongst other names, depending on the country, honeydew honey is sweet, dark, strong, and sticky, and processed by honey bees and stingless bees from a sugar-rich tacky liquid secreted by aphids and some scale insects as they feed on plant saps.

Some of the plants from which bees collect honeydew include silver fir, spruce, Greek fir, pine, hazel, maple, ash, apple, black beech, red beech, apricot, willow, rowan, linden, American elm, citrus, white poplar, holm oaks, chestnut, cork oaks, plum, peach, alfalfa, and others. Insect sources include wood and plant lice (also known as blackflies, greenflies, or whiteflies), *Metcalfa pruinosa*, scale insects, some moths and caterpillars, but aphids are the main insects.

The majority of the plants that are attacked by these flies are trees, the coniferous trees yielding the highest amounts of honeydew worldwide. However, cotton, alfalfa, sunflower, and other plants can also provide honeydew and from these honey bees elaborate honeydew honey.

Honeydew honey is less sweet and darker than regular honey, crystallization rate is slow, and its taste and aroma tend to be resinous, woody, or spicy.

Honeydew honey is high in polyphenolic compounds, flavonoids, minerals, amino acids, quinoline alkaloids, trisaccharides and other oligosaccharides, and it contains pollen, mold hyphae and spores, and unicellular algae.

Its main biological properties are: a very high antioxidant, antifungal, antibacterial, pain-soothing (antinociceptive), gastroprotective, and prebiotic activity. It improves memory, inhibits *Helicobacter pylori*, the causing agent of gastritis and peptic ulcers, preserves the gastric mucosa capillaries, boosts mucous production, and has a very high antiradical scavenging activity.

An excellent online article on honeydew honey (theresearchpedia.com/health/superfoods) describes these and other biological activities of honeydew or forest honey and its potential role in Apitherapy:

- Its value as prebiotics: oligosaccharides present in honeydew serve as prebiotics promoting the growth of beneficial bacteria present in the gut. It is very helpful if consumed after taking antibiotics that are generally used to treat bacterial infections. By improving the gut flora, it even helps to increase appetite.

- It supports free radical elimination: a high concentration of antioxidants in this honey variety helps with the elimination of free radicals and reduces the damage caused by them. Thus, intake of honeydew honey promotes general health.

- Antibacterial action: the honeydew variety of honey serves as a powerful antibiotic due to the presence of high glucose oxidase activity. Its high enzymatic action results in the production of increased amounts of hydrogen peroxide which in turn acts against bacteria. Apigenin and kaempferol play an important role in honeydew honey antibacterial action. In fact, it serves as an antibacterial agent even stronger than manuka honey which is renowned for its superior antiseptic qualities. Being an antibacterial agent, it also serves as a perfect remedy for cough.

- Nourishing the nervous system: its high concentration of amino acids and minerals such as cobalt, manganese, zinc, phosphorus and sulphur helps in nourishing the nervous system. It even benefits in the improvement of cerebral functions. By improving the cerebral functions, intellectual abilities are heightened.

- Due to the presence of high amounts of mineral salts, it serves as substitute for the sodium typically integrated in sports drinks. Dissolve one to two spoons of honeydew honey in a glass of water to obtain the desired salts. This property of honeydew makes it a better drink even for athletes looking to improve performance.

- It is very delicious in taste and is best enjoyed as a spread for stale bread and toasts.

- It improves the taste of cheese varieties such as Gorgonzola, Murianengo, Roquefort, and Taleggio.

Regrettably, to this date, honeydew honey has limited availability in markets, daily life use, and Apitherapy practice despite its virtues.

3.9 MEAD

Mead has tens or perhaps hundreds of versions according to the recipe used: traditional mead includes only honey, yeast, and water, and its taste resembles Chardonnay or Riesling wines. Melomel is a mead with added fruit such as grapes (pyment), apples (cyser), blackberry, raspberry, strawberry, or malted barley and hops (braggot or bracket). Metheglin and hypocras are meads elaborated with added flavors from herbs and spices like vanilla, jasmine, lavender, meadowsweet, ginger, tea, orange peel, chamomile, coriander, cloves, nutmeg, cinnamon, and others. Cinnamon or vanilla are often components of melomels, metheglin, and hypocras. As it happens with wines, there are so many recipes, types, and brands of mead that expert have compiled many books on the subject.

Most of biological properties known for honey are also valid for mead. An excellent mead is made from *zabrus* (honeycomb capping).

Bees have lactic acid in their stomachs that, mixed with honey, could cure chronic wounds in animals that had previously resisted other types of treatment. It fights resistance to antibiotics, has antibacterial, antifungal, and antiviral action, antioxidant, and cicatrizing properties.

AN EASY MEAD RECIPE

The following mead recipe is very simple and it belongs to the Savannah Bee Company, in Georgia, USA, who has generously shared it online with you in the website https://savannahbee.com/blog/making-honey-mead-1-gallon-tupelo-dry-traditional-mead/ . I immediately loved it because it uses tupelo (*Nyssa* sp.) honey, my favorite one and the most popular honey in northwest Florida, USA. You will need:

- Two one-gallon (3.8 liters each) glass jugs. This can be a carboy from a homebrew shop or as easy as the jug that apple juice comes in. You will need one for primary fermentation and a second to transfer to for aging.

- Thermometer.

- Hydrometer (optional). This is also purchased at a homebrew shop or online. It measures the specific gravity, which is the density of your mead. With this tool, you will be able to figure out the final alcohol by volume (ABV).

- Airlock. This piece is essential. It allows the carbon dioxide created by the yeast to escape without oxygen getting in. It also lets you monitor the fermentation.

- Racking cane and tubing. You will use it to transfer the mead from your primary to the secondary fermenter vessel (glass jug).

Once fermentation is complete you will want to bottle the mead. For this I recommend:

- Four 750 mL glass bottles, four corks, one funnel, and one bottle corker.

Ingredients:

- One kilogram of tupelo honey (you can use any honey you like), three liters of water, one package of champagne yeast or wine yeast.

Preparing the must takes only about thirty minutes.

- Wash the glass jug or carboy with warm to hot water and dish soap.

- Pour the water and honey into the container. Mix until the honey is dissolved in the water.

- If you have a hydrometer, place it in the honey water and take a reading. It resembles a floating thermometer. Note where the floating piece rests. This is your original gravity. Write it down. Later you will compare it to the reading you get post fermentation to determine the ABV.

- Heat half a cup of water to 40 degrees Celsius. Add the package of yeast. Stir until thoroughly mixed and let it stand for fifteen minutes.

- Pour your water-yeast mixture into the honey-water mix or must.

- Shake the glass container to mix the yeast into the honey water. This adds oxygen to begin the fermentation process.

- Now, plug the jug with the airlock. Additional oxygen is not your friend! Place the jug in a cool dry place away from sunlight.

- Now you wait. After about a day you should notice bubbles in the airlock. This is how you know you are successful and fermentation has begun. If fermentation is quite slow (less than one bubble in the airlock per minute) you may wish to add the additional honey as a yeast nutrient. After about a month it is time to transfer the fermenting must to the second container. You are welcome to taste it at this point by syphoning off some with the racking cane. Transferring the must removes it from the spent yeast that has fallen to the bottom of the container and leads to a clearer mead.

- Place the carboy/jug with the fermenting must on a table. Place the second container on the floor below.

- Remove the airlock and place the racking cane inside and lead the tube to the second container. Siphon the must into your second container, letting gravity do most of the work.

- Place the airlock into the second container and move it back to your cool, dry, dark storage place.

- Watch the airlock. Once the bubbles stop completely fermentation has been accomplished. Remove it and you may measure the gravity again using your hydrometer. This is known as the final gravity. Write it down. Then use an ABV calculator, such as the one found at brewersfriend.com, to determine the ABV. It should fall in the standard strength mead range, which is 7.5 – 14 %.

Now you can taste the mead. It will probably taste too "sharp" at this point. You'll want it to condition in bottles for anywhere from one month to a year. This is where the four bottles come in handy. Open one after a month, the second three months later, and so on. Take notes, and remember what worked best for the next time you make mead.

- Wash your bottles and funnel with water and dish soap.

- Fill your bottles using the funnel and cork them using the bottle corker.

- Store in a refrigerator. Mead is best stored at cellar temperature, just like wine. If you have a wine cellar or cool basement, great! Otherwise, place the bottles in temperature controlled refrigerator that you dial to 7 – 10 degrees Celsius. You may wish to chill the mead in the refrigerator before serving.

3.10 MELIPONA HONEY

O f the 20,000 known bee species, stingless bees account for more than 500 species, and most belong to only three genera.

Mayan mead was called *acan*: since hundreds of years prior to Spanish conquer of western hemisphere, Central American Mayans used to prepare *acan*, a fermented drink from stingless bee honey (*kab*), sometimes with the addition of fruits or corn.

The common names most known for stingless bees are abeja real, alazán, borá, canche, chelerita, congo, congo negro, criolla, culo de chucho, doncellita prieta, erica, guanota, homo, jandaira, jataí, jolocán, madaçaia, mosquito, negrita, pegoncito, pisil nekmej, pringador, serenita, taxcat, tenchalita, tinzuca, tiúba, uruçu and many other denominations to all the stingless bees or specifically to *Melipona*, *Scaptotrigona*, or *Trigona* species.

This honey is extracted with syringes as it is extremely fluid (up to 30 % water), clear like white morning glory (*Rivea corymbosa*) honey, and it has high acidity (maximum 70 - 85 meq/100 mg), a minimum of 50 g reducing sugars per 100 g honey, diastase activity minimum 3.0 in *Melipona* and *Scaptotrigona*, 7.0 in *Trigona*; sucrose maximum 6 g/100 g for *Melipona* and *Trigona*, 2 g/100 g for *Scaptotrigona*; and water content up to 30 g/100 g

Melipona honey has a high price and its therapeutic uses include the treatment of bruises, casts for fractures, delivery enhancer, digestive disorders, ear pain, eye diseases, cataracts, conjunctivitis, pterygium, fatigue, head external injuries, post-birth recovery, respiratory infections, skin ulcers, stomach disorders, aches, and wound healing.

3.11 POLLEN

The best food ever known and the most complete source of proteins or essential amino acids in Nature is bee pollen. No animal or plant food has all essential amino acids, almost all vitamins, more than eight flavonoids, growth regulators, auxins, gibberellins, cytokinins, nucleic acids, microelements like magnesium, calcium, iron, and phosphorus, enzymes, and other bioactive substances. It is the only known nutrient for prostate health, and one kilogram of pollen contains three times more protein than one-kilogram of beef.

It is used as a dietary supplement during recuperation periods, in cases of malnutrition, asthenia and apathy, and to increase physical and mental ability or strengthen the immune system. It prolongs one's life span, promotes weight gain, increases plasma hemoglobin levels, and provides tissues with vitamin C and Mg thanks to its active substances, including amino acids, vitamins like tocopherol, niacin, thiamine, biotin, and folic acid. In a study in 1946, it was found that most of 100-year-old and older Georgian/Russian people used to eat bee pollen. To consume, it is best to dissolve two or three tablespoons of pollen into one glass of water for 15 – 20 minutes.

Pollen has anti-inflammatory, anticholesterolemic, immunoprotecting, antiproliferative, wound healing, anti-ulcerous, hepatoprotective, antianemia, relaxing, radioprotectant, and other properties.

As pollen and apitoxin are highly allergenic, make sure to perform allergy tests before use to prevent anaphylaxis.

Bee pollen is used in complementary and alternative medicine to cure prostatitis, stomach ulcers, infectious diseases, and for the prevention and treatment of high-altitude-sickness syndrome. A wide range of therapeutic properties have been suggested, including antimicrobic, antioxidant, hepatoprotective, chemopreventive and anticarcinogenic, antiatherosclerotic, anti-inflammatory, antiallergenic, and immune modulatory activities.

The antioxidant property of bee pollen seems to be mainly due to phenolic acids, like vanillic, protocatechuic, gallic, and p-coumaric acids, and to flavonoids like hesperidin, rutin, kaempferol, apigenin, luteolin, quercetin, and isorhamnetin. These compounds are thought to inactivate electrophiles and scavenge free radicals and reactive oxygen species.

Its antimicrobial effects against Gram-positive and Gram-negative pathogenic bacteria, microscopic fungi/yeasts are mediated by glucose oxidase activity, deriving from honeybee secretion, while plant phenolics and flavonoids could also be involved.

Its anti-inflammatory effects have been compared to those of common non-steroidal anti-inflammatory drugs, possibly depending on the activity of flavonoids, phenolic acids, phytosterols, and flavoring substances like anethole. Pollen also has the capability of removing swellings caused by cardiovascular and renal pathologies, of protecting the liver from carbon tetrachloride-induced damages, and of alleviating prostate inflammation and hyperplasia. Positive effects on prostatic conditions have been also ascribed to antiandrogen actions.

Bee pollen has potential anticancer activity, probably associated with its antioxidant and antimutagenic potentials. It has antiatherosclerotic and cardioprotective effects and it has been successfully applied to patients who did not respond to classical drugs. Pollen's hypolipidemic activity is attributed to the presence of unsaturated fatty acids, especially the ω-3,α-linolenic acid (a major inhibitor of platelet aggregation), and to phospholipids and phytosterols. It has antidiabetic compounds in pollen grains, such as steroids, alkaloids, saponins, flavonoids, sugars, tannins, suggesting therapeutic possibilities for bee pollen as a hypoglycemic agent.

To collect 200 g of pollen (less than a cup), a single worker bee would need to perform 13,400 flights for a total of 40,000 km: a circumferential trip around our planet. Subsequently, bees collect pollen from plants which is then mixed with their salivary secretions and nectar, and bring it back to the hive packed into pellets and stored in the combs by other worker bees as the protein food for the colony.

3.12 PROPOLIS

I n 1979, propolis was called "the purple gold of bees" (in *Propóleo, un valioso producto apícola*, and later in *Propóleo, el oro púrpura de las abejas*, and other books) because red propolis resembles Tyrian purple or royal purple. But more accurately, however, it should be called "the burgundy gold of bees" or else, as propolis's hues from black, brown, burgundy, green, yellowish, and other colors depending on its plant source. In fact, although hive air, honeydew honey, mead, bee bread, drone larvae, and other hive products are valuable and are used mainly in 21st century, neither one of these products is as amazing as propolis, which unfortunately has been beekeeping's and Apitherapy's "Ugly Duckling" or "Cinderella".

Bees need sun, air, water, carbohydrates, proteins, and defense substances to live. Honey acts as the carbohydrate, pollen as the protein, and propolis as the all-spectrum antibiotic and defense substance for a bee colony.

Propolis is a resinous, sticky material collected by foraging bees from plant exudates, mucilage, resins, lattices, gums, and buds (50 %) and mixed with bee enzymes and wax (30 %), plus 10 % essential oils, 5 % pollen, and 5 % other substances. It is used by bees in the hive as a protective substance or sanitizer and a compact, malleable building material. If any small or big enemy such as a rat or a snake intrudes in a hive, worker bees go into counteroffensive mode and furiously sting it to death, embalming the intruder's corpse immediately afterwards. The propolis-embalmed mummy can remain intact for hundreds of years, just like ancient Egyptian mummies stay preserved to this day thanks to propolis. This valuable resin was used in ancient times as an ingredient in healing formulas used by ancient Egyptian priests thousands of years ago, and thus womb-like aseptic conditions inside the hive do not become damaged in time.

The chemical composition of propolis is dramatically dependent on its geographical and floral origins. Raw propolis generally contains more than 300 different compounds, mostly consisting of triterpenes (50 % w/w), waxes (25 – 30 %), volatile mono- and sesquiterpenes (8 – 12 %), giving propolis its typical resinous odor, and phenolics (5 – 10 %). European and Asian propolis contain simple phenolic acids, while lignans are main compounds in tropical propolis. Other types of propolis's common constituents include: organic acids, ketones, aldehydes, hydrocarbons, minerals, benzoic acid, benzyl alcohol, vanillin, eugenol, phenolics compounds, flavonoids, phenolic acids, flavonoid aglycones and esters of substituted cinnamic acids.

The biological activities of propolis are amazing: strong anesthetic, fastest wound/burn healer, antibacterial and other antimicrobial, antifungal, antiviral, cytotoxic, antioxidant, anti-inflammatory, immunomodulatory, anxiolytic, anticancer, among others. It acts simultaneously against antibiotic-resistant bacteria, fungi, and viruses. It contains secondary plant metabolites, including volatiles and up to 10 % volatile oils, and they have an antioxidant, antifungal, antibacterial and other antimicrobial activity. Caffeic acid phenethyl ester is perhaps the most important compound in American, European, and Asian propolis, while Brazilian green propolis (derived from exudates and resins of South American alecrim-do-campo or tula, *Braccharis dracunculifolia*) is characterized by the presence of 3,5-diprenyl-4-hydroxycinnamic acid, artepillin C, together with other prenylated cinnamic acids and caffeic acid derivatives.

Propolis is a very safe product, non-toxic and well tolerated. However, there is no information on LD_{50} in humans. It is documented that in mice and rats, LD_{50} exits as 7.34 g/body kg, thus in humans it could be 587 g for an 80-kg person. No observed adverse effect level is over 1470 mg/kg/day or 118 g a day for six months for a person weighting 80 kg. Despite its favorable safety profile, propolis is a common cause of allergic reactions, and It has been reported that 1.2 – 6.6 % of patients with dermatitis are sensitive to propolis, while its major sensitizers are 3-methyl-2-butenyl caffeate, phenylethyl caffeate, benzyl salicylate, benzyl cinnamate, and 1,1-dimethylallylcaffeic acid.

Pinobanksin-3-acetate has been indicated as the strongest antioxidant constituent of propolis. Caffeic acid phenethyl ester has anticancer properties including prostate cancer, breast cancer and human immunodeficiency virus, while artepillin C has antiproliferative properties. Propolis is the bee product containing the highest amount of phenolics and thus it has been deeply studied for its antioxidant and radical scavenging activities. Several of these compounds possess strong antioxidant and antiradical activities, including pinocembrin, chrysin, and pinobanksin.

Propolis possesses antibacterial properties against Gram-positive and Gram-negative strains, including methicillin-resistant *Staphylococcus aureus*, vancomycin-resistant *Enterococci*, *Helicobacter pylori*, and *Streptococcus* sp., and thanks to the presence of such flavonoids as galangin, pinocembrin, rutin, quercetin, and naringenin, and caffeic acid phenethyl ester, since these compounds increase bacterial membrane permeability. Galangin, pinocembrin, and caffeic acid phenethyl ester inhibit bacterial RNA polymerase. The antimicrobial activity of Brazilian red propolis depends on its peculiar content in isoflavones. Antibacterial effectiveness has been demonstrated in different propolis volatile fractions, including β-eudesmol, δ-cadinene, α-pinene, trans-β-terpineol, β-eudesmol, benzyl benzoate, nerolidol, spatulenol, ledol, farnesol, dihydroeudesmol, and guaiol. The antibacterial property of Brazilian propolis has been revealed in its volatile fractions containing nerolidol, spatulenol, p-cimen-8-ol, ethylphenol, β-caryophyllene, acetophenone, α-pinene, β-pinene and limonene.

This valuable bee resin acts as an antifungal agent against pathogenic yeasts like *Candida albicans*, *C. parapsilosis*, *C. tropicalis*, and *C. glabrata*. Antifungal activity has been also shown in volatile compounds from Brazilian propolis, viz. α-pinene, β-pinene and δ-cadinene, phenyl-, ethyl-, and benzyl alcohol, and decanal. The ethanolic extracts of propolis have strong anti-*Candida albicans* activity imputable to the inhibition of germ tube development by phenolic, aromatic, and aliphatic acids. An ethanolic extract containing caffeic acid phenethyl ester and other caffeic acid derivatives is effective against *Candida albicans*, *C. dubliniensis*, *C. glabrata*, *C. krusei*, *C. parapsilosis*, and *C. tropicalis*, like red Brazilian propolis is rich in triterpenes and isoflavones, such as formononetin, medicarpin, and vestitol.

Propolis is well known for its antiviral activity, which in some cases can exceed that of standard drugs. A propolis ointment has better results than acyclovir in the clinical treatment of genital herpes simplex. Antiviral properties seem to depend mainly on the presence of caffeic acid phenethyl ester and related compounds. Caffeic acid phenethyl ester inhibits the activity of HIV by acting on viral integrase, and suppresses the hepatitis C virus. Propolis containing caffeic acid derivatives is effective on herpes simplex virus; 3,4-dicaffeoylquinic acid, a major constituent of Brazilian green propolis, represses influenza A virus by upregulating the apoptosis-inducing ligand.

The bee resin is rich in phenolic acids and flavonoids and possesses antiproliferative and proapoptotic properties. Components such as chrysin, galangin, caffeic acid phenethyl ester, benzyl ferulate, benzyl isoferulate, pinostrobin, 5-phenylpenta-2,4-dienoic acid, tectochrysin, artepillin C, pinobanksin, pinobanksin-3-O-propanoate, pinobanksin-3-O-butyrate, pinobanksin-3-O-pentanoate, polycyclic, polyisoprenylated benzophenone nemorosone cardanol and cardol exert an antiproliferative and proapoptotic effect on several human cancer cells of lymphoma, breast, colorectal, prostate, lymphoblastic leukemia cancers, esophageal squamous cancer, and gastric carcinoma.

Propolis modulates immune responses, and this kind of impact could explain to some extent its antimicrobial and antiviral activities. Brazilian green propolis standardized in 18.9 % w/w polyphenols, 9.85 % flavonoids and 2.3 artepillin C improves phagocytosis, the production of antibodies against erythrocytes, and ear swelling.

It has strong anti-inflammatory properties, possibly linked to the presence of phenolic acids, mainly caffeic acid phenethyl ester.

Propolis is the finest and fastest wound healer in Nature, better than aloe and other plant resins. A mouth sore heals within 24 hours of propolis application and a gastroduodenal ulcer heals in 15 days, the same as any infected open wound. Its healing effect on diabetic foot ulcers is well known, as is other problematic tissue injuries, and it is favored by the immunomodulatory, antioxidant and antiseptic effects of this resin regurgitated by bees from plant resins and other plant parts. Propolis modulates fibronectin expression and collagen deposition in burns. Brazilian green propolis, rich in artepillin C, has revealed superior wound healing activity with respect to Brazilian red propolis.

Main sources of propolis are tola or alecrim-do-campo (*Braccharis dracunculifolia*), avocado (*Persea americana*), *Clusia rosea*, black poplar (*Populus nigra*), oak (*Quercus robur*), horse-chestnut (*Aesculus hippocastanum*), pine (*Pinus* sp.), dalbergia (*Dalbergia ecastophyllum*), birch (*Betula* sp.), alder (*Alnus glutinosa*), hazel (*Corylus avellane*), Antilles calophyllum (*Calophyllum antillanum*), turpentine tree (*Bursera simaruba*), guaguasí (*Zuelania guidonia*), *Cistus clusii*, balsam apple (*Clusea major*), manajú (*Rheedia aristata*), mango (*Mangifera ndica*), and red mangrove (*Rhizophora mangle*).

3.13 ROYAL JELLY

In 1792, Swiss naturalist François Huber appointed the name of royal jelly to the secretion of honeybee hypopharynx and mandibular salivary glands, however previously, in 1586, Spanish Luis Méndez de Torres had found that the queen bee is of the female sex and the mother and ruler of the bee colony. Royal jelly is a white-yellowish, gelatinous, acidic colloid, composed of about 67 % water (w/w), 16 % sugar, 12.5 % protein and amino acids, and 5 % fat, with considerable variability among different sources. Minor royal jelly constituents include enzymes, vitamins, phenolics, and minerals. Proteins are the most abundant dry matter fraction, consisting of more than 80 % of soluble glycoproteins named major royal jelly proteins. Its main ingredients comprise the 10-carbon atoms fatty acids trans-10-hydroxy-2-decenoic acid, unique to royal jelly, and 10-hydroxydecanoic acid. Sterols are also present in minor amounts.

Royal jelly is also fed by nurse bees until the third day of life to larvae developing into female workers (sterile, they live 30 - 90 days and weigh 125 mg) and male drones (fertile, they live 28 - 62 days until their fatal nuptial flight and all survivors are sacrificed by worker bees, and weigh 277 - 290 mg), or until the end of the larval period to selected individuals developing into queens (fertile, the survivor lives six years and weighs 240 mg; all other pretenders are sacrificed by worker bees). Moreover, it is an exclusive food for adult queens throughout their life. The induction of larval development into queen has been ascribed to major royal jelly proteins, and it is essential for the breeding of royal larvae which gain 1500 times their weight in 16 days until reaching their complete evolution as queens.

Royal jelly has been used since ancient times in traditional medicine, especially in Asian Apitherapy, but also in the ancient Egypt. It is currently used in the pharmaceutical and cosmetic fields, and marketed as an over-the-counter nutritional supplement. It has antiseptic activities against bacteria, fungi and viruses. It is also hypotensive, collagen boosting, antitumor, antihypercholesterolemic, antiaging, anti-inflammatory, antidiabetic properties, positive effects on benign prostatic hyperplasia, and wound healing of diabetic foot ulcers and other wounds, contains gamma globulin, estradiol, testosterone, progesterone, and acetylcholine. Small peptides consisting of 2 – 4 amino acid residues possess its strong antioxidant activity. Most active ones have tyrosine residues at the C-terminal, allowing hydroxyl radical and hydrogen peroxide scavenging activities.

Despite its multiple therapeutic and nutritional applications, royal jelly must be taken in small amounts to prevent cephalgia, artery pressure increase, cardiac rhythm increase, and nausea. The recommended dose is 100 - 300 mg (a teaspoon), and no more than 500 mg daily intake is recommended. Royal jelly consumption can occasionally lead to contact dermatitis, asthma and anaphylaxis, while trans-10-hydroxy-2-decenoic acid and 10-hydroxydecanoic acid have been identified as major allergens.

Royalisin is an amino acid peptide, homologous to the hemolymph defensin-1, with antibacterial activity against various Gram-positive strains, including *Staphylococcus, Streptococcus, Bacillus subtilis, Micrococcus luteus, Sarcina lutea, Clostridium, Corynebacterium, Lactobacillus helveticus, Paenibacillus larvae*, and Leuconostoc, while no inhibition has been observed against the Gram-negative *Escherichia coli* and *Serratia marcescens*. Antifungal activity against *Botrytis cinerea* has also been reported for royalisin. Apalbumin inhibits the growth of *Pseudomonas larvae, Bacillus subtilis*, and *Escherichia coli*. Royal jelly carboxylic acids collectively exert antimicrobial properties against Gram-positive, Gram-negative bacteria, and fungi. Trans-10-hydroxy-2-decenoic acid is a particularly strong antibacterial compound, especially against *Bacillus subtilis, Staphylococcus aureus*, and *Escherichia coli*. Correspondingly, sebacic acid has strong antifungal activity against *Candida albicans, C. tropicalis*, and *C. glabrate*.

Trans-10-hydroxy-2-decenoic acid and 4-hydroperoxy-2-decenoic acid ethyl ester protect from gastric ulcer, inhibit fibroblast-like synoviocytes from rheumatoid arthritis patients, and inhibit histone deacetylase activity, and have therapeutic potential against atherosclerosis.

The royal jelly proteins possess bile acid-binding properties and increases hepatic cholesterol catabolism. Trans-10-hydroxy-2-decenoic acid enhances insulin-independent muscle glucose uptake and improves the hyperlipidemic condition. Royalactin and trans-10-hydroxy-2-decenoic acid extend the lifespan of honey bees.

Royal jelly has estrogen-like effects and acts as an anti-menopause agent, ascribed to the ability of lipids trans-10-hydroxy-2-decenoic acid, trans-2-decenoic, 10-hydroxydecanoic, 3,10-dihydroxydecanoic, and sebacic acids, and steroid 24-methylenecholesterol to act as weak activators of estrogen receptors. Trans-10-hydroxy-2-decenoic acid promotes collagen synthesis and the production of the collagen promoting factor, transforming growth factor β1, in human skin fibroblasts.

Trans-10-hydroxy-2-decenoic acid and 10-hydroxydecanoic acid have shown to stimulate neuron differentiation from rat embryo's neural stem cells, possibly acting like the ω-3 docosahexaenoic acid, an essential diet component that is known to promote neurogenesis in the central nervous system. Docosahexaenoic acid is reputed essential for brain development and function and has shown positive results in Parkinson's disease, suggesting similar potentials for trans-10-hydroxy-2-decenoic acid, which could cross more easily the blood-brain barrier due to its smaller molecule. The neurogenerative potentials of royal jelly fatty acids are also suggested as 2-decenoic acid ethyl ester, a derivative of the royal jelly 2-decenoic acid, which promotes functional recovery of spinal cord injuries.

3.14 WHOLE BEES

Whole bees are a valuable food for birds and poultry and for that reason chickens and other birds are seen seeking for dead bees close to hives. In winter, beekeepers find many dead bees on the bottom of hives which are being collected by researchers to study their medicinal properties once those bees are dried and lyophilized.

The bodies of bees are surrounded with a hard integument-cuticle, which serves to support the internals and as protection from external threats. There are outgrowths which form on the cuticle with muscles fastened to them. All the diversity of the integument creates in the process of the insect development by means of cells that make cuticle. The cells have cubical and cylindrical shapes forming a thick layer called hypoderm. The cuticle is very solid but flexible thanks to chitin. The percentage of chitin in the cuticle is from 30 % to 50 %. Chitin makes cuticle elastic and its hardness and impenetrability is provided by its complicated structure.

In the cuticle of insects, chitin is covalently bound to melanins and sclerotin-like proteins, forming compounds that undergo considerable degradation during their separation. Chitosan and triturated whole bees have been used for many years in ancient pharmacopeias. Their nutritional value is well known by beekeepers who also share their profession with poultry farming.

The processing of whole bees includes trituration, drying or lyophilization. Some preparations also include a deproteinization of bees with a 10 % alkaline solution and deacetylation with a 50 % NaOH solution at 125 ± 50 degrees Celsius. The procedure of isolation of chitin, chitosan, and water-soluble low-molecular-weight chitin from the corpses of bees includes deproteinization of the corpses of bees, discoloration of the chitin-melanin complex, deacetylation, and enzymatic hydrolysis of chitosan.

Whole bees are rich in chitosan, a polymer of β-(1-4)-D-glucosamine and N-acetyl-β-D-glucosamine (deacetylated unit) and N-acetyl-D-glucosamine (acetylated unit), very abundant in the exoskeleton of crustaceans, and with very interesting medicinal properties. This polymer was discovered in 1811 in France by Henri Braconnot. Chitosan is made by treating the chitin shells of bees, shrimp and other crustaceans with an alkaline substance, like sodium hydroxide. Lyophilized whole bees or chitosan have been shown to reduce blood cholesterol levels and the body absorption of fat and carbohydrates. It also improves blood microcirculation and intestinal peristalsis, reduces toxin contact with intestinal walls, reduces toxin penetration in blood stream, normalizes intestinal function and gastrointestinal tract microflora, and helps the body eliminate excess chlorine and sodium. It is an indigestible substance (fiber) which binds various fat in the large intestine and thereby blocks its absorption. As a result, cholesterol levels decrease, reducing high blood pressure and the risk of cardiovascular diseases. It reduces appetite and improves the function of the large intestine. Chitosan also absorbs toxins and contaminants in the body therefore furthering the process of body detoxification.

It limits fat absorption in the body, inhibits duodenal absorption and enhances lipid excretion. As a soluble dietary fiber, it may increase gastrointestinal lumen viscosity and delay the emptying of the stomach, creating a sense of satiety. It alters bile acid composition, increasing the excretion of sterols and reducing the digestibility of ileal fats. Lyophilized whole bees or chitosan allow to rapidly clot blood, and has recently gained approval in the US and Europe for use in bandages and other hemostatic agents as chitosan is hypoallergenic, has natural antibacterial and hemostatic properties, and reduces pain by blocking nerve endings.

3.15 *ZABRUS* OR HONEYCOMB CAPPING

There is a 15th bee product mentioned by some apitherapists: *zabrus* or **забрус** (a Russian word meaning "sealant caps" or "honeycomb capping" in English, and "opérculos" in Spanish) is a cut strip of the upper lids of sealed honeycombs, "highly effective in the treatment of bacterial and viral diseases of nasopharynx and upper respiratory tract, it does not cause allergies, chewing of *zabrus* is useful in many ways: it causes severe salivation, which increases the secretion and gastric motility" (http://keepingbee.org/honey-bee-products/), and in wounds, infections, and other respiratory disorders. Ancient people chewed the seal of bees as a hygienic remedy for teeth and gum problems.

Honeycomb capping are stored with honey at room temperature or without honey in the refrigerator, always light protected. It is used for chewing gums, suppositories, cosmetics, lotions, and ointments.

It's antibacterial and antiviral thanks to its lysozyme. It activates and strengthens the metabolic processes and blood circulation, as well as the intestinal peristalsis, acting as a mild laxative for intestinal cleansing and fecal obstruction.

Use it for bruises and wound healing, has anti-inflammatory and local anesthetic properties, it is used for sinusitis, sore throats, severe acute respiratory syndrome, asthma allergic rhinitis, and activates salivary glands. It can be ingested in moderate doses, or to chew one teaspoon of *zabrus* four to seven times a day for, 15 minutes each time.

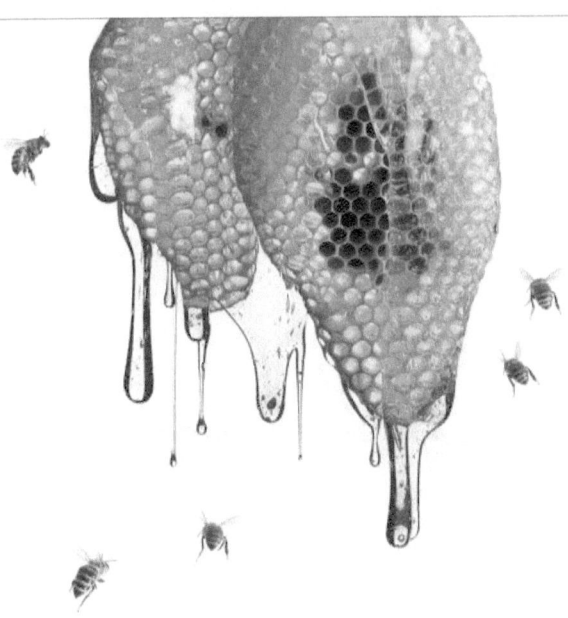

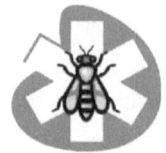

4. INFORMED CONSENT FOR APITHERAPY

Héodore Cherbuliez (1927 - 2016), MD, who was President and Vice-President of the American Apitherapy Society (AAS), President of the Swiss Apitherapy Society, and President of the Apitherapy Commission of Apimondia, used to remark the importance of clinical documentation for the practice of Apitherapy and all kind of therapies, and he was one of the designers of the AAS informed consent for Apitherapy treatment and suggested the use of health evaluation forms, treatment logs, progress notes, body diagrams, and other clinical tools.

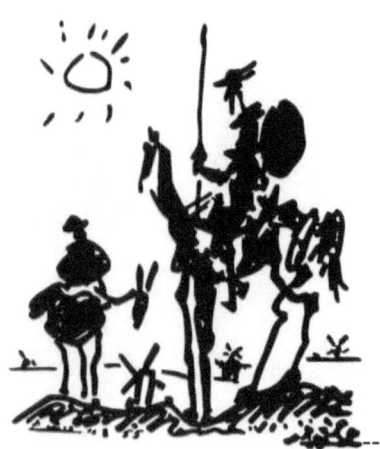

Apitherapy, Sancho, in 20th and 21st centuries there will be a new revolution for Complementary and Alternative Medicines. Apitherapists are altruist and cost-benefit effective practitioners for most health problems in the world. They shall be honored by a Moisés Asís hence in this book as 'the new Quixotes and Sanchoes of Healing Arts'.

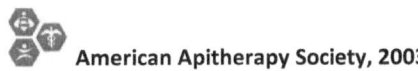

INFORMED CONSENT FOR APITHERAPY TREATMENT

American Apitherapy Society, 2003

APITHERAPY is the art and science of making therapeutic use of products of the beehive, such as honey, bee pollen, bee bread, propolis, géopropolis, Melipona honey, whole bees, mead, honeydew honey, royal jelly, beeswax, honeycomb capping, hive air, drone larvae, and bee venom. Maximum effectiveness depends, on a relationship of trust and confidence between the Apitherapist and the recipient of APITHERAPY, called here the Client. Both parties must recognize the need to cooperate and work together to deal with such facts as stated below:

I, the Client, understand that:

APITHERAPY addresses the whole body, including mind and spirit, in a holistic way;

* APITHERAPY is not a treatment approved by the US Food and Drug Administration, the American Medical Association, or any other regulatory or recognized scientific body in the United States;

* There are not clearly established protocols for APITHERAPY treatments;

* Complications of APITHERAPY include itching, swelling, bruising, infection, temporary increase in pain, and allergic reactions ranging from skin irritation or rash up to anaphylactic shock and death;

* Honeybee stings are painful.

The Apitherapist has advised me of the procedure planned. I have received a clear, comprehensive explanation of the risks inherent in this APITHERAPY treatment and their possible adverse consequences, including death. I have discussed these matters with the Apitherapist and am satisfied that the briefing has been understandable and thorough and that it adequately addressed my concerns. I am confident that I have the information necessary to understand the risks and benefits of the procedure so I may give this informed consent.

The Apitherapist has made no warranties, guarantees, or promises of any kind regarding the safety or efficacy or results of the treatment.

I have given the Apitherapist a clear, candid, and complete disclosure of my relevant medical history, including problems, treatments, and medications. (For instance, bee stings cannot safely be given to persons taking beta blockers, since they render ineffective the antidote to anaphylactic shock, the principal risk of bee venom treatment.) Should I begin to exhibit signs of a significant allergic reaction, I authorize the Apitherapist to administer epinephrine and/or an antihistaminic.

I have been informed that alternatives to APITHERAPY may include surgery, medication, massage, spinal manipulation, medical treatment and advice, and a regimen of diet and exercise All have been considered, and I have chosen to pursue APITHERAPY for relieving pain, enhancing well-being, and/or improving my physical   condition.

By signing this agreement, I give this informed consent to receive APITHERAPY treatment and I release the Apitherapist from liability for any harm which it may cause me and I covenant not to sue in the event of an ineffective, inadequate, or adverse result (meaning no change or a worsening of my condition). I understand that I am entitled to receive a copy of this consent form when it is executed.

I, the Apitherapist, state that I have fully and frankly explained the risks and benefits of APITHERAPY and pledge my best efforts to administer it in a proper manner based on my training, experience, and best judgment.

WHEREFORE, In consideration of their mutual undertakings, and in reliance on their reciprocal obligations, both Apitherapist and Client represent that they have read and understood this document, affirm the statements they make above and evidence their acceptance of the above terms by signing below.

Signed and sealed this _____day of_____,20__ at _____

Client _____   Apitherapist _____

CONSENTIMIENTO INFORMADO PARA APITERAPIA

(Traducido/adaptado de *JAAS* 10(1):9, 2003 para *Apiterapia 101 para todos*)

APITERAPIA es el arte y ciencia de hacer uso terapéutico de los productos de la colmena, tales como la miel, polen de las abejas, propóleo, jalea real, larvas de zángano, miel de meliponas, geopropolis, pan de abejas, aire de la colmena, opérculos, hidromiel, miel de rocío, abejas enteras, cera y veneno de abejas. La efectividad máxima depende en gran parte de la relación de confianza entre el Apiterapeuta y quien recibe la APITERAPIA, llamado aquí el Cliente. Ambas partes deben reconocer la necesidad de cooperar y trabajar juntos en lo siguiente.

Yo, el Cliente, entiendo que:

•La APITERAPIA afecta a todo el cuerpo, incluyendo mente y espíritu, en forma holística;

•La APITERAPIA no es un tratamiento aún aprobado por las instituciones médicas, reguladoras o científicas oficialmente reconocidas en el país;

•No existen protocolos establecidos claramente para los tratamientos de APITERAPIA;

•Las complicaciones de la APITERAPIA incluyen erupciones, inflamación, moretones, infección, aumento temporal del dolor y reacciones alérgicas que van desde irritación o erupción cutánea hasta choque anafiláctico y muerte;

•Las picaduras de abejas son dolorosas.

El Apiterapeuta me ha explicado el procedimiento previsto. Yo he recibido una explicación clara y general de los riesgos inherentes en este tratamiento de APITERAPIA y sus posibles consecuencias adversas, incluyendo la muere. Yo he discutido estos temas con el Apiterapeuta y estoy satisfecho(a) de que la explicación ha sido comprensible y completa y que ha respondido adecuadamente a mis dudas. Confío en que tengo la información necesaria para entender los riesgos y beneficios del procedimiento, de modo que yo pueda dar mi consentimiento.

El Apiterapeuta no me ha dado garantías o promesas de ningún tipo acerca de la seguridad, eficacia o resultados del tratamiento.

Le he dado al Apiterapeuta toda la información clara, sincera y completa sobre mi historia clínica, incluyendo problemas, tratamientos y medicamentos. (Por ejemplo, no pueden aplicarse picaduras de abejas con seguridad a personas que estén tomando ß-bloqueadores, ya que hacen inefectivo el antídoto al choque anafiláctico, principal riesgo del tratamiento con veneno de abejas.) En caso de que yo empiece a manifestar signos de reacción alérgica significativa, autorizo al Apiterapeuta a administrar epinefrina, antihistamínicos o ambos.

He sido informado(a) que las alternativas a la APITERAPIA pueden incluir cirugía, medicación, masaje, manipulación de la columna vertebral, tratamiento y consulta médica, así como un régimen de dieta y ejercicio. Pese a tener conocimiento de estas alternativas, he elegido proseguir con la APITERAPIA para aliviar el dolor, tener mayor bienestar o mejorar mi condición física.

Mediante la firma de este acuerdo, doy este consentimiento para recibir tratamiento de APITERAPIA y libro al Apiterapeuta de responsabilidad por cualquier daño que pueda causarme y me comprometo a no demandarlo en caso de un resultado inefectivo, inadecuado o adverso (lo que significa ningún cambio o empeoramiento de mi condición). Entiendo que estoy en el derecho de recibir una copia de este modelo de consentimiento cuando sea ejecutado.

Yo, el Apiterapeuta, afirmo que he explicado completa y francamente los riesgos y beneficios de la APITERAPIA y dedicaré mis mejores esfuerzos a administrarla de modo apropiado en base a mi entrenamiento, experiencia y buen juicio.

POR TANTO, en consideración de sus compromisos mutuos y en base a sus obligaciones recíprocas, Apiterapeuta y Cliente señalan que ambos han leído y comprendido este documento, afirman las declaraciones que han realizado y evidencia su aceptación de los anteriores términos firmando a continuación.

Firmado y sellado este día _____ del mes de _____ de 20___, a la hora_____ en _____ ☘

Cliente: _____

Apiterapeuta: _____ _____

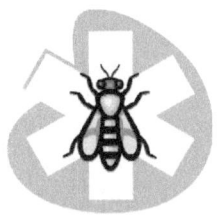

5. MEDICAL ASSESSMENT

Also known as health history, medical history, health assessment, clinical history, among others, characterizes all the available clinical information on the patient including his/her demographic information, past and present health conditions, interventions, allergies, active medications including beta-blockers and other contraindications in the case any chance of anaphylactic reaction occurs, as well as all pertinent documentation on the person. The medical assessment, informed consent form, body chart, allergy form, medication log, progress notes, SOAP form, Apipuncture meridians, and any other documentation, should be filed together in the client's record. Several different forms of each category have been included for your convenience and may use the as needed.

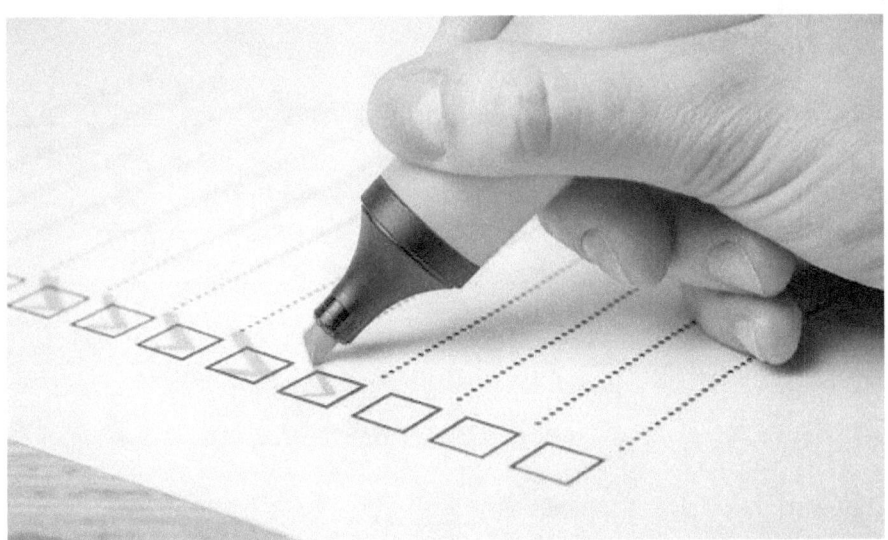

Health Assessment Form

Name: _____ Date of Birth: _____

Gender: _____ Employee No. _____ Position: _____

Street Address: _____

_____

City: _____ State: _____ Zip: _____

Telephone: _____ Email: _____ Fax: _____

I. Medical conditions

Heart Failure   _____ Hypertension _____

Angina   _____ Hypercholesterolemia _____

Emphysema   _____ Asthma _____

Allergic rhinitis   _____ Diabetes _____

Thyroid disease   _____ Esophagitis _____

Duodenal, stomach or Peptic ulcer _____ Glaucoma _____

Original Date:
Dates Revised:

HEALTH ASSESSMENT FORM

All questions contained in this questionnaire are strictly confidential
and will become part of your medical record.

Name (Last, First, M.I.)		☐ M ☐ F	DOB:
Marital status: ☐ Single ☐ Partnered ☐ Married ☐ Separated ☐ Divorced ☐ Widowed			
Previous or referring doctor:		Date of last physical exam:	

PERSONAL HEALTH HISTORY

Childhood illness:	☐ Measles ☐ Mumps ☐ Rubella ☐ Chickenpox ☐ Rheumatic Fever ☐ Polio	
Immunizations and dates:	☐ Tetanus	☐ Pneumonia
	☐ Hepatitis	☐ Chickenpox
	☐ Influenza	☐ MMR Measles, Mumps, Rubella

List any medical problems that other doctors have diagnosed

Surgeries

Year	Reason	Hospital

Other hospitalizations

Year	Reason	Hospital

Have you ever had a blood transfusion?	☐ Yes ☐ No

Date	Mode of Arrival	Medic Unit ____	Pain Scale:	PMD:	TRIAGE CATEGORY
	☐ Walk ☐ W/C ☐ Gurney ☐ Carried ☐ Police		0 1 2 3 4 5 6 7 8 9 10		I II III IV V

RAPID ASSESSMENT

Does the patient have an infection or suspicion of infection? Yes No   Is patient on antibiotics (not prophylaxis?) Yes No

CHIEF COMPLAINT:

AIRWAY	BREATHING	CIRCULATION	NEURO	Time of Assessment: ____
☐ Patent	☐ Unlabored	☐ Palpable pulse ____	☐ Alert ☐ Oriented ☐ Confused	Rapid Triage RN Signature:
☐ Impaired	☐ Labored	☐ Strong ☐ Weak ☐ Regular ☐ Irregular	☐ Unresponsive	
	☐ Shallow ☐ Deep	☐ Normal ☐ Pale ☐ Jaundice ☐ Cyanotic	☐ Clear ☐ Slurred ☐ Garbled	

TEMP oral	PULSE	RESP	BP	Rt	Sat Rm Air -RA	ACCUCHECK	WEIGHT : KG STATED ACTUAL	Ht	IMMUNIZATION	LMP	ROOM	TIME	PLACED IN RM BY
rectal:				Lt									

ALLERGIES: (Drug / Reaction) ☐ NKDA

Glasgow Coma Scale			PAIN SCALE: 0 1 2 3 4 5 6 7 8 9 10	☐ See Medication Reconciliation Form HISTORY	
			On Arrival ____	☐ None ☐ Substance Abuse ☐ Sz	
Best Eye Opening	4 - Spontaneous	2 - To pain	PAIN: Onset ____	☐ CVA ☐ ETOH ☐ Psych	
	3 - To voice	1 - None	Location: ____	☐ Cardiac ☐ COPD ☐ Dialysis	
Best Verbal	5 - Oriented (Coos, babbles)	2 - Incomp. sounds	**INTERVENTION**	☐ Diabetes ☐ Asthma Last Tx ____	
	4 - Confused (cries)	1 - None	☐ Ice ☐ Elevate ☐ Soft splint	☐ HTN ☐ GI ☐ Unknown	
	3 - Inappr words (screams/grunts)		☐ Dressing applied ☐ Bleeding controlled	☐ Smoker ☐ GU ☐ Migraines	
Best Motor	6 - Obeys commands (Spont.)	3 - Flexion	☐ Hard Collar placed ☐ Acetaminophen	☐ Elevated Cholesterol ☐ Breast Feeding	
	5 - Localizes pain	2 - Extension	☐ NPO instruction given ☐ Ibuprofen	☐ CA ☐ Thyroid	
	4 - Withdrawal	1 - None	☐ Respiratory Precautions Initiated	☐ Other ____	
			VISUAL ACUITY		
GCS Total:			LT RT BOTH CORRECTED ☐ YES ☐ NO		

PRE HOSPITAL CARE VS: P____ R____ BP____ SPO2____ /O2____ L/min	SKIN SIGNS	GAIT: ☐ Steady ☐ W/Crutches/Cane
Cardiac Rhythm ____ C-spine precautions ☐ Yes ☐ No	☐ Normal, Warm , Dry	☐ In W/C ☐ Not Observed ☐ ____
Respiratory Assist ☐ Yes ☐ No ETT ☐ Yes ☐ No CPR ☐ Yes ☐ No	☐ Cyanotic ☐ Clammy	RME MD/PA/NP: ____
Accucheck ____ Medication/Treatments ____	☐ Pale ☐ Diaphoretic	Time of Assessment ____
IV ☐ Yes ☐ No	☐ Jaundice ☐ Hot	Comprehensive Triage/ Assessment RN Signature
Gauge ____ Site ____	☐ Flushed ☐ Cool	

NEURO		EXTREMITY C.S.M. ☐ N/A	CARDIOVASCULAR ☐ N/A	RESPIRATORY ☐ N/A	
☐ ALERT	☐ RESTLESS	**CAPILLARY REFILL**	**PULSES**	☐ SYMMETRICAL ☐ ASYMMETRICAL	
☐ ORIENTED	☐ COMBATIVE	Rt Arm ____ Rt Leg ____	☐ STRONG ☐ JVD	RESPIRATIONS LUNG SOUNDS	
☐ COOPERATIVE	☐ CRYING	Lt Arm ____ Lt Leg ____	☐ REGULAR ☐ PEDAL EDEMA	☐ UNLABORED LT RT	
☐ CLEAR	☐ SLURRED	**SENSATION**	☐ IRREGULAR	☐ LABORED ☐ CLEAR ☐	
☐ UNCONSCIOUS	☐ GARBLED	Rt Arm ____ Rt Leg ____		☐ SHALLOW ☐ WHEEZES ☐	
☐ SEE NEURO FLOW SHEET		Lt Arm ____ Lt Leg ____	**PEDIATRICS**	☐ DEEP ☐ RALES ☐	
		MOVEMENT / STRENGTH	CAPILLARY REFILL ____	☐ RETRACTION ☐ RHONCHI ☐	
		Rt Arm ____ Rt Leg ____	FONTANEL ____	☐ NASAL FLARING ☐ DIMINISHED ☐	
☐ PUPILS ☐ N/A		Lt Arm ____ Lt Leg ____	# OF WET DIAPERS ____ x 24	☐ ACCESSORY MUSCLE USE	
Size: Rt ____ Lt ____		W - weak D - delayed over 2 sec.		☐ ABSENT ☐	
Reactivity: Rt ____ Lt ____		A - absent N - numbness	TEARS ____	☐ PAINFUL ☐ COUGH	
		T - tingling P - painful B - brisk		☐ ABSENT SPUTUM COLOR	
		II - irregular I - intact	MUCOUS MEMBRANES ____	☐ MECHANICAL/SUPPORTED ____	

GI / GU ☐ N/A		SKIN INTEGRITY	SCREENING TOOL		
ABDOMEN	**INCONTINENCE**			NON-CONTRIBUTORY	REFERRAL
☐ UNREMARKABLE	☐ BOWEL		NUTRITION ____	☐	☐
☐ SOFT	☐ BLADDER		DOMESTIC VIOLENCE ____	☐	☐
☐ FIRM	☐ CATHETER PRESENT		PSYCHOSOCIAL ____	☐	☐
☐ DISTENDED	**GENITALS**		SKIN INTEGRITY ____	☐	☐
☐ TENDER	☐ DISCHARGE: COLOR		EDUCATION ____	☐	☐
☐ NONTENDER			COMMUNICATION BARRIER ☐		
☐ PAINFUL	☐ BLEEDING		INTERPRETER ____		
☐ MASSES	____ MAXI PAD/____ HR		INTERVENTION ____		
☐ RIGID	____ MINI PAD/____ HR				
☐ REBOUND	____ TAMPON/____ HR				
☐ NAUSEA	☐ OTHER ____		☐ Sepsis/Aspiration screen completed		
☐ VOMITING x ____	Gravida ____ Para ____				
☐ DIARRHEA x ____	TAB ____ SAB ____				
BOWEL SOUNDS	EDC ____ FHT ____	A - Abrasion FB-Foreign Body S - Swelling	Patient Identification		
☐ PRESENT	☐ Dysuria	B - Burns H - Hematoma 1 - Stage I			
☐ ABSENT	☐ Hematuria	C - Redness P - Pain/Tender 2 - Stage II			
☐ HYPOACTIVE		D - Deformity L - Laceration 3 - Stage III			
☐ HYPERACTIVE	LAST BM ____	E - Ecchymosis PW-Puncture Wound 4 - Stage IV			
		F - Edema R - Rash 0 - Other			

ASSESSMENT RN SIGNATURE ____ **Time:** ____

☐ Assessment completed by RME MD/PA/NP Time: ____

09993 (5/31/98)

HISTORIA CLÍNICA

Nombre:_____ _____
_____ Sexo____Edad_____ Ocupación_____
_____
Motivo de Consulta_____
Antecedentes Personales Patológicos.
(Detallara los antecedentes de importancia clínica, así como el tratamiento que recibe para cada situación comórbida y su duración)

Cardiovasculares____
Pulmonares____
Digestivos_____
Diabetes___ Renales_____
Quirúrgicos_____
Alérgicos_____
Transfusiones____
Medicamentos_____
Especifique_____ _____
_____ _____
_____

Antecedentes Personales No Patológicos
(se anotará aquí lo relacionado a tabaquismo, uso de alcohol, así como diferentes adicciones y su duración, de igual forma se anotarán aquí, de requerirse, los antecedentes sexuales del paciente.)

Alcohol: _____
Tabaquismo: _____
Drogas: _____
Inmunizaciones: _____
Otros:

_____ _____
_____

Antecedentes Familiares:

Padre: Vivo Si____ No____ Enfermedades que padece:_____
_____ _____
_____ _____

Madre: Viva Si____ No____ Enfermedades que padece:_____
_____ _____
_____ _____
_____

Hermanos: ¿Cuántos?_____Vivos____Enfermedades que padecen:
_____
_____ _____
_____ _____
_____

Otros:
_____ _____
_____

Antecedentes Gineco-obstétricos:
Menarquia_____ Ritmo _____ F.U.M._____ G___ P____ A_____ C_
_____ I.V.S.A_____ Uso de Métodos Anticonceptivos: Si _____ No _____
__ ¿Cuáles?_____
_____

Enfermedad Actual
del Paciente _____
____ _____ __
_____ _____
_____ _____
_____ _____
_____

Exploración física.

Signos Vitales
TA
(brazo derecho)

TA
(brazo izquierdo)

F.C_____Frec. Resp._____Temp._____Peso_____Talla_____IMC_____

Cabeza y
Cuello_____

_____ _____

Tórax_____

_____

Abdomen. _____

_____

_____

Extremidades. _____

_____

Neurológico y Estado
Mental _____

🐝 HEALTH ASSESSMENT FORM

Client Name_____

Date_____ Session #_____

S:_____
_____
O:_____
_____
_____
A:_____
_____
P:_____

Date_____ Session #_____

S:_____
_____
O:_____
_____
_____
A:_____
_____
P:_____

Date_____ Session #_____

S:_____
_____
O:_____
_____
_____
A:_____
_____
P:_____

Date_____ Session #_____

S:_____
_____
O:_____
_____
_____
A:_____
_____
P:_____

Final Notes:_____

HEALTH ASSESSMENT FORM

COMPANY: _____

DOCTOR: _____

DATE: __/__/____

Name:

PAN:

Date:

Primary:

Secondary:

Record:

Diagnosis	Procedures

Subjective:

Objective:

Assessment:

Plan:

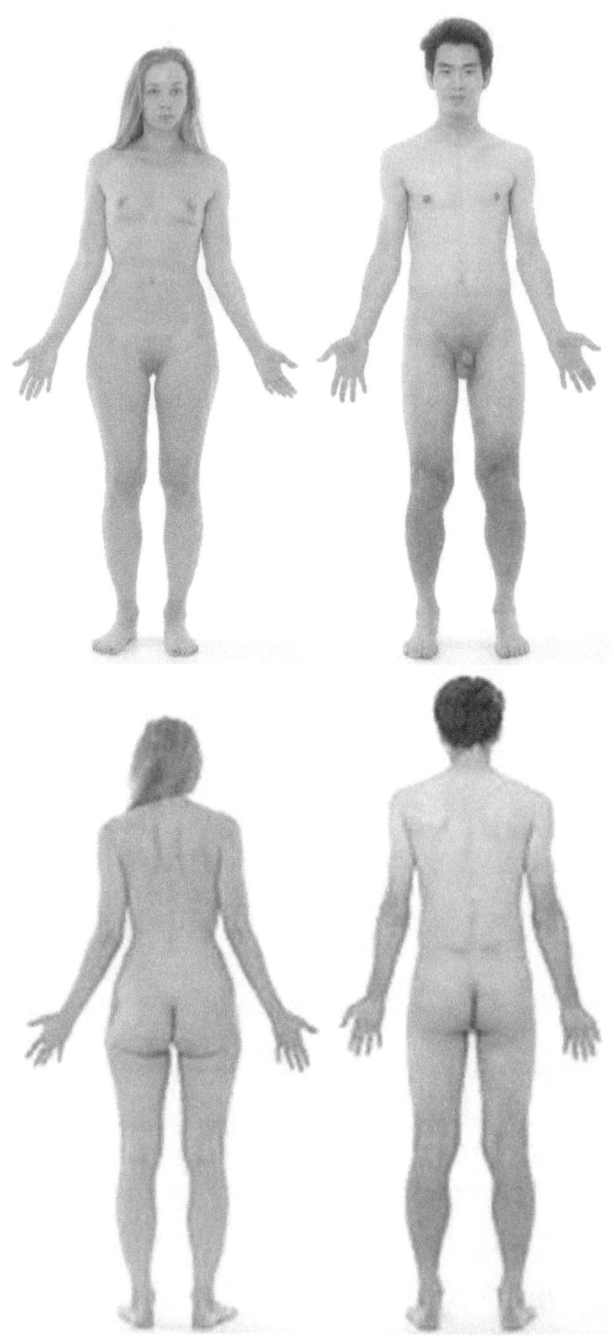

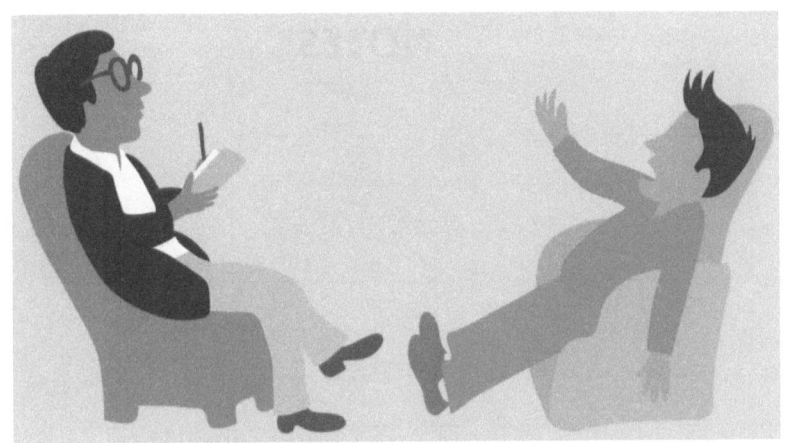

-- DOCTOR ANN MARY, 9 YEARS AGO YOU PROGNOSED MY LIFE EXPECTANCY WOULD BE 8 MORE MONTHS DUE TO AN AGGRESSIVE CANCER. BUT IN FACT, THANKS TO PROPOLIS, BEE VENOM THERAPY AND OTHER APITHERAPY PRODUCTS, THERE WAS APOPTOSIS OF CANCER CELLS AND I HAD A 99 % REMISSION.

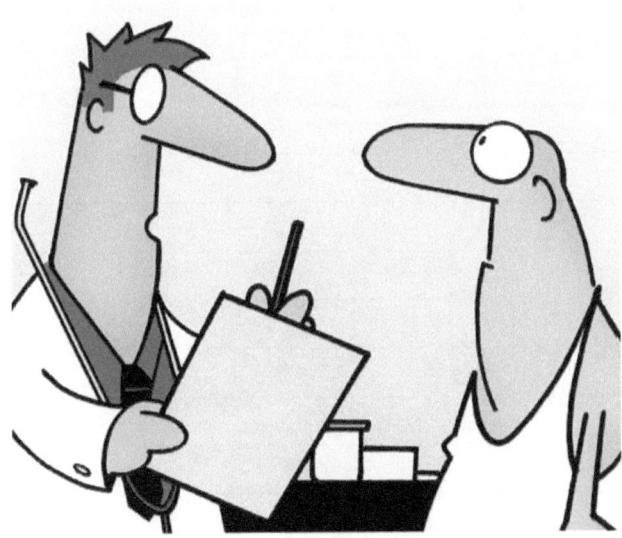

-- SEÑOR ALEX, YOU HAVE A HEART CONDITION AND MUST IMMEDIATELY STOP VIAGRA FOR YOUR E.D.; BUT THE GOOD NEWS IS THAT, IN LIEU OF IT, FROM NOW ON, I WILL PRESCRIBE PROPOLIS DROPS AND BEE BREAD FOR YOU.

NOTES

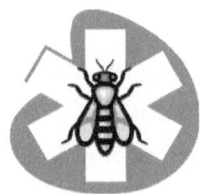

6. MEDICATION LOG

t's very important to know what medications and treatments the client is taking.

The use of beta blockers is contraindicated for the use of bee venom or apitoxin and any bee product thus risking an anaphylactic reaction in the patient.

Herein a list of main beta-blockers and a list of abbreviations commonly used in prescription medications.

This list could be much longer with the addition of new products and multiple brand names used in different countries. Generic names for the main component are in parenthesis. For any question, search in updated drug reference manuals or online in any of the several websites such as www.pdrhealth.com, www.drugs.com, www. rxmedsguide.com, www.rxlist.com and others.

BETA-BLOCKERS / Betabloqueadores

IMPORTANT: Never use apitoxin (bee venom) if beta-adrenergic blocking drugs (ß–blockers) are being taken. Best known ß–blockers and their combinations are:

- Ablok (Atenolol)
- Ablok Plus (Atenolol)
- Acebutolol
- Angipress-CD (Atenolol)
- Antitensin (Propanolol HCl)
- Apo-Atenolol (Atenolol)
- Apo-Metoprolol (Metoprolol tartrate)
- Apo-Propanolol (Propanolol HCl)
- Apo-Timol (Timolol maleate)
- Atenalon (Atenolol)
- Ateneo (Atenolol)
- Atenol (Atenolol)
- Atenolol
- Atenopress (Atenolol)
- Atenoric (Atenolol)
- Atepress (Atenolol)
- Betacar (Betaxolol HCl)
- Beta-cardone (Sotalol HCl)
- Betaloc (Metoprolol tartrate)
- Betapace (Sotalol HCl)
- Betaxolol HCl
- Betim (Timolol maleate)
- Betoptic (Betaxolol HCl)
- Biconcor (Bisoprolol fumarate)
- Bisoprolol fumarate
- Blocadren (Timolol maleate)
- Brevibloc (Esmolol HCl)
- Cardicor (Bisoprolol fumarate)
- Cardilol (Carvedilol)
- Cardiopranol (Propanolol HCl)

- Carteolol HCl
- Cartrol (Carteolol HCl)
- Carvedilol
- Celectol (Celiprolol HCl)
- Celiprolol HCl
- Concor (Bisoprolol fumarate)
- Coreg (Carvedilol)
- Corgard (Nadolol)
- Dilatrend (Carvedilol)
- Divelol (Carvedilol)
- Esmolol HCl
- Eucardic (Carvedilol)
- Inderal (Propanolol HCl)
- Inderal-LA (Propanolol HCl)
- Inderide (Propanolol HCl)
- Inderide-LA (Propanolol HCl)
- Kerlone (Betaxolol HCl)
- Labetalol HCl
- Levatol (Penbutolol)Levobunolol
- Lopressor (Metoprolol tartrate)
- Metipranolol
- Metoprolol tartrate
- Monitan (Acebutolol)
- Monocor (Bisoprolol fumarate)
- Nadolol
- Nebilet (Nebivolol)
- Nebivolol
- Neo Propranol (Propanolol HCl)
- Normodyne (Labetalol HCl)
- Novo-Atenolol (Atenolol)
- Novometoprol (Metoprolol tartrate)
- Novo-Pindol (Pindolol)
- Novo-Timol (Timolol maleate)
- Ocupress (Carteolol HCl)
- Oxprenolol HCl
- Penbutolol
- Pindolol

- Plenacor (Atenolol)
- Propranolol Ayerst (Propanolol HCl)
- Propranolol HCl
- Rebaten la (Propanolol HCl)
- Sectral (Acebutolol)
- Seloken (Metoprolol tartrate)
- Selopress (Metoprolol tartrate)
- Selozok (Metoprolol tartrate)
- Sotacor Sotalol HCl)
- Sotalol HCl
- Tenadren (Propanolol HCl)
- Tenoretic (Atenolol)
- Tenormin (Atenolol)
- Teoptic (Carteolol HCl)
- Timolol maleate
- Timoptol (Timolol maleate)
- Toprol-XL (Metoprolol tartrate)
- Trandate (Labetalol HCl)
- Trasicor (Oxprenolo HCl)
- Viskaldix (Pindolol)
- Visken (Pindolol)
- Zebeta (Bisoprolol fumarate)

ABBREVIATION USED IN PRESCRIPTION

Abbreviation	Latin	Meaning
• aa	ana	of each
• ac	ante cibum	before meal
• ad	-	to, up to
• a.d.	aurio dextra	right ear
• ad lib.	ad libitum	use as much as one desires, freely
• agit. ante us	agita ante usum	shake before taking
• alt. h. (alt hor)	alternis horis	every other hour
• a.m.	ante meridiem	morning, before noon
• amp	-	ampule
• amt	-	amount
• aq	aqua	water
• a.l., a.s.	aurio laeva, aurio sinister	left ear
• A.T.C	-	around the clock
• a.u.	auris utrae	both ear
• b.i.d	bis in die	use twice a day
• bis	bis	twice
• B.M.	-	bowel movement
• bol.	bolus	a large pill
• B.S.	-	body surface area
• c	cum	with
• cap., caps.	capsula	capsule
• c	cibos	food
• cc	-	cubic centimeter, also means "with food" (cum cibos)
• cf	-	with food
• D5W	-	dextrose 5% solution
• D5NS	-	dextrose 5% in normail saline
• D.A.W.	-	dispense as written
• dc, D/C, disc	-	Discontinue
• dieb. alt	diebus alternis	every other day
• dil.	-	dilute
• disp.	-	dispense

73

MEDICATION LOG

Name   :

Date of Birth   :

Address   :

SSN   :

Doctor   :

Doctor Phone #   :

Pharmacy   :

Pharmacy Phone #   :

Medication	Dosage	Date	Time	Remark

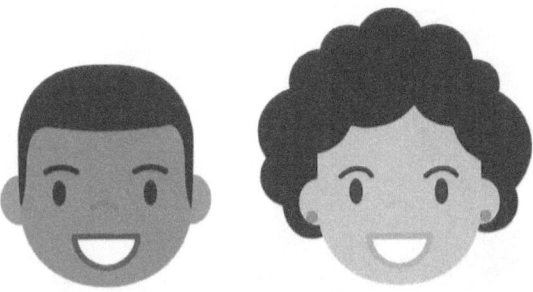

-- AS YOU KNOW, KATHERINE, BIG PHARMA AND PREDATORY MEDICINE PRICES ARE HURTING MANY PEOPLE...

-- YES, BUT THANK HEAVEN, **WE APITHERAPISTS CAN HEAL A WHOLE COMMUNITY** FOR ONLY PENNIES. EVERY HUMAN BEING HAS ACCESS TO HONEY, PROPOLIS, APITOXIN, BEE OLLEN, HIVE AIR, ROYAL JELLY, BEESWAX, DRONE LARVAE, AND ALL OTHER BEEHIVE PRODUCTS.

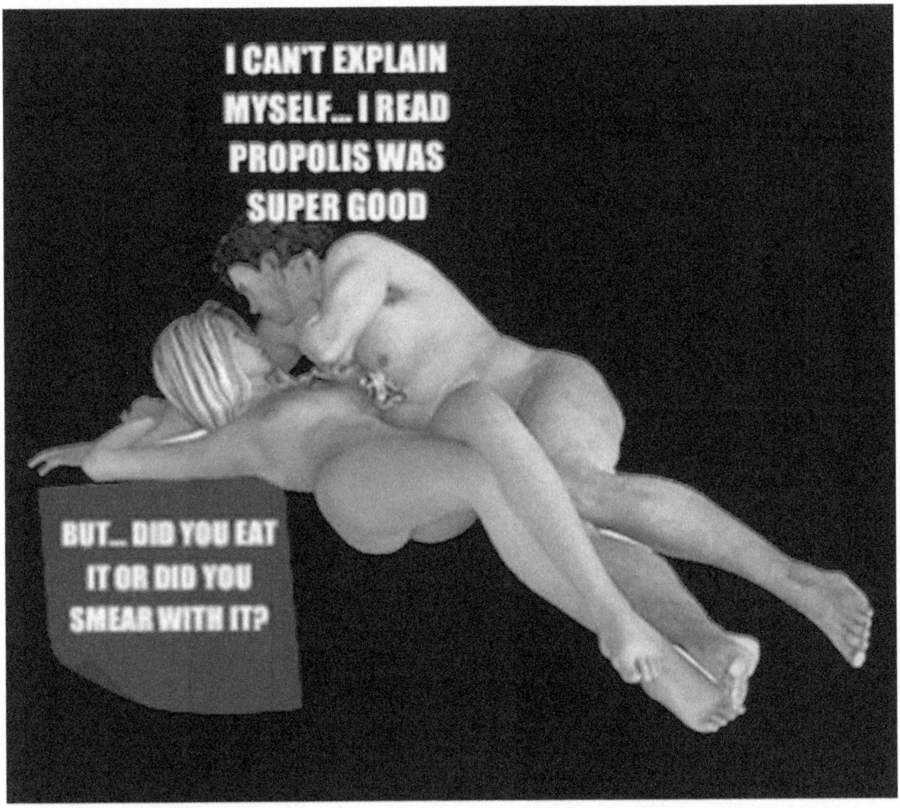

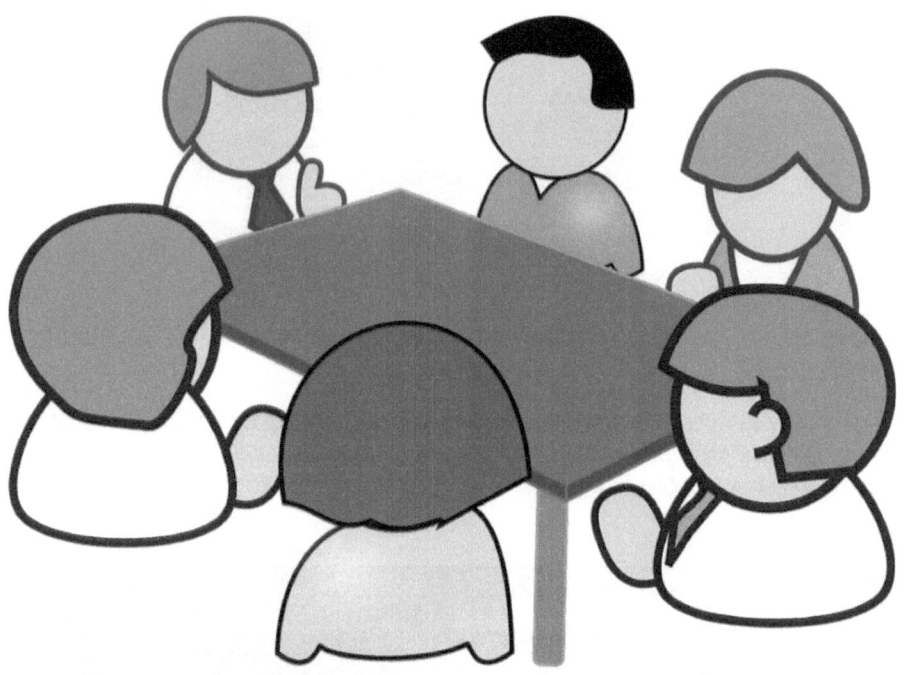

DURING AN UNDATED APITHERAPEUTIC BOARD MEETING IN THE FICTICIOUS REPUBLIC OF SOUTH GWANDANOLAND:
-- MANUKA, TUALANG, OR KANUKA HONEY PATCHES?
-- NO, BETTER TO APPLY RED OR GREEN PROPOLIS ON IT.
-- I'D RATHER RUB WITH BEE VENOM OINTMENT! AND HONEYCOMB CAPPING.
-- IN MY OPINION, BEE BREAD OR GÉOPROPOLIS WILL HEAL IT.
-- MELIPONA HONEY AND HONEYDEW HONEY ARE ALSO GREAT FOR IT.
-- BUT MEAD WILL EVENTUALLY HEAL IT AND WILL MAKE EVERYBODY VERY HAPPY, AND IT'S CHEAPER!

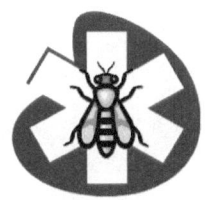

7. NOTES ON ALLERGIES

| 1 | Have a written emergency protocol for recognition and treatment of anaphylaxis and rehearse it regularly. |

| 2 | Remove exposure to the trigger if possible, eg. discontinue an intravenous diagnostic or therapeutic agent that seems to be triggering symptoms. |

| 3 | Assess the patient's circulation, airway, breathing, mental status, skin, and body weight (mass). |

Promptly and simultaneously, perform steps 4, 5 and 6.

| 4 | Call for help: resuscitation team (hospital) or emergency medical services (community) if available. |

| 5 | Inject epinephrine (adrenaline) intramuscularly in the mid-anterolateral aspect of the thigh, 0.01 mg/kg of a 1:1,000 (1 mg/mL) solution, maximum of 0.5 mg (adult) or 0.3 mg (child); record the time of the dose and repeat it in 5-15 minutes, if needed. Most patients respond to 1 or 2 doses. |

🐝 ## ALLERGY AND SYMPTOM TABLE

SYMPTOMS

Check all that apply

	Runny Nose	Scratchy Throat	Hives	Itching	Rash	Facial Swelling	Facial Color	Cramping
Shellfish								
Peanuts	√				√			
Eggs								√
Wheat								
Soy				√				√
Beer		√						
Alcohol								
Dyes			√					
Milk								
Antibiotics			√					
Pain Meds						√		
Anesthetics								
Dust							√	
Mold								

ALLERGY LOG

	Rash	Itching	Hives	Constipation	Diarrhea	Hard to Breathe	Cramping	Scratchy Throat	Runny Nose	Facial Color	Swelling
ANIMALS											
Cats											
Dogs											
Insects											
Other											
MEDICATIONS											
Antibiotics											
Pain Medication											
Anesthetics											
Other											
ENVIRONMENT											
Dust											
Mold											
Cleaning Products											
Pollen											
Grasses											
Trees											
Other											
FOODS											
Shellfish											
Peanuts											
Eggs											
Wheat											
Soy											
Other											
DRINKS											
Beer											
Other Alcohol											
Juice											
Milk Products											
Other											

ALLERGY EMERGENCY ACTION PLAN

ID: _____Student Name:_____ Birthdate: _____

Teacher/Grade: _____

Parents/Guardians: _____

Contact Information: (H) _____ (C) _____
                          (W) _____ (C) _____

Physician Name: _____ Physician Phone: _____

Allergy to: _____

Weight: _____lbs.　Asthma: ☐ Yes (higher risk for a severe reaction) ☐ No

Extremely reactive to the following foods:_____
THEREFORE:
☐ If checked, give epinephrine immediately for ANY symptoms if the allergen was *likely* eaten.

☐ If checked, give epinephrine immediately if the allergen was *definitely* eaten, even if no symptoms are noted.

Any SEVERE SYMPTOMS after suspected or known ingestion:

One or more of the following:
LUNG:	Short of breath, wheeze, repetitive cough
HEART:	Pale, blue, faint, weak pulse, dizzy, confused
THROAT:	Tight, hoarse, trouble breathing/swallowing MOUTH: Obstructive swelling (tongue and/or lips) SKIN: Many hives over body

Or combination of symptoms from different body areas: SKIN: Hives, itchy rashes, swelling (e.g., eyes, lips) GUT: Vomiting, crampy pain

➡

1. **INJECT EPINEPHRINE IMMEDIATELY**
2. Call 911
3. Begin monitoring (see box below)
4. Give additional medications:*
   -Antihistamine
   -Inhaler (bronchodilator) if asthma

*Antihistamines & inhalers/bronchodilators are not to be depended upon to treat a severe reaction (anaphylaxis). USE EPINEPHRINE.

MILD SYMPTOMS ONLY:

MOUTH:	Itchy mouth
SKIN:	A few hives around mouth/face, mild itch
GUT:	Mild nausea/discomfort

➡

1. **GIVE ANTIHISTAMINE**
2. Stay with student; alert healthcare professionals and parent
3. If symptoms progress (see above), USE EPINEPHRINE
4. Begin monitoring (see box below)

Medication/Doses
Epinephrine: Brand_____Dose_____
Antihistamine: Brand_____Dose_____
Other (e.g., inhaler-bronchodilator if asthmatic): _____
Self-Administration (Pupil has the discretion as to the use of his/her medication)
(   ) Yes　*I certify that the above named student has been instructed in the use and self-administration of
_____. He/she understands the needs for the medication and the
necessity to report to school personnel so that 911 can be called.

ALLERGY EMERGENCY ACTION PLAN

NM FOOD/INSECT & EMERGENCY ALLERGY ACTION PLAN and MEDICATION AUTHORIZATION

School District / School Name _____ Date _____

Student Name	Date of Birth	Student #	
*Health Care Provider Name/Title	Provider's Office Phone / FAX #		Place student's picture here
Parent/Guardian	Parent's Phone #s		
Emergency Contact	Contact Phone #s		

Known Life-Threatening Allergies:

History of Asthma? ☐ No ☐ Yes
(Asthma may indicate an increased risk of severe reaction)

Diagnosis of Mild Allergy? ☐ No ☐ Yes
Please list allergens:

History of SEVERE Anaphylactic Reaction? ☐ No ☐ Yes,
If checked YES, give epinephrine immediately!
Give epinephrine if allergen was likely eaten, at onset of any symptoms or if allergen was definitely eaten even if no symptoms are noticed.

TREATMENT PLAN

FOR ANY OF THE FOLLOWING SEVERE SYMPTOMS:

LUNG:	Difficulty breathing or swallowing, wheezing, coughing
HEART:	Dizzy, faint, confused, pale, blue, weak pulse
THROAT:	Tight, hoarse, trouble breathing/swallowing, drooling
MOUTH:	Significant swelling of tongue, lips
SKIN:	Many hives over body, widespread redness over body
GUT:	Nausea, repetitive vomiting, severe diarrhea, cramping
Other:	Feeling something bad is about to happen, anxiety, confusion

FOLLOW THIS PROTOCOL:
1. INJECT EPINEPHRINE IMMEDIATELY! (Note time)
2. Call 911. Request ambulance with epinephrine.
3. Don't hang up & don't leave student
4. Give additional medications as ordered
   - Antihistamine (if ordered below)
   - Inhaler (Albuterol) if student has asthma
5. Lay student flat and raise legs. If breathing is difficult or vomiting, sit up or lie on their side
6. Notify School Nurse and Parent/Guardian
7. Notify Prescribing Provider / PCP
8. Student must be transported to ER

☐ **MILD ALLERGY SYMPTOMS IF DIAGNOSIS CONFIRMED ABOVE:**

MOUTH:	Itchy mouth, lips, tongue and/or throat
SKIN:	Itchy mouth
NOSE:	Itchy/runny nose
GUT:	Mild nausea/discomfort

1. GIVE ANTIHISTAMINE as directed
2. Monitor student; alert emergency contacts
3. Watch student closely for changes
4. If symptoms worsen, GO TO EPINEPHRINE PROTOCOL (see above)

THE SEVERITY OF SYMPTOMS CAN QUICKLY CHANGE. ALL SYMPTOMS OF ANAPHYLAXIS CAN POTENTIALLY PROGRESS TO A LIFE THREATENING SITUATION!

MEDICATION ORDER

Epinephrine	☐ Epinephrine (0.15mg) inject intramuscularly	☐ Epinephrine (0.3mg) inject intramuscularly
Student's weight ____ lbs.	EpiPen Auvi Q Adrenaclick	EpiPen Auvi Q Adrenaclick
	A second dose of epinephrine can be given 5 minutes or more after the first if symptoms persist or recur.	

Antihistamine	☐ Benadryl/Diphenhydramine	☐ Other _____	SIDE EFFECTS OF EPINEPHRINE MAY INCLUDE:
Do not depend on antihistamines (or inhalers). When in doubt, give epinephrine and call 911.	Dose: Route: PO Frequency:	Dose: Route:	ANXIETY, TREMOR, PALPITATIONS, DIZZINESS, WEAKNESS, TINGLING, & PALENESS

NOTE: IF NURSE IS NOT AVAILABLE, THE ABOVE TREATMENT PLAN MAY BE PROVIDED BY TRAINED SCHOOL PERSONNEL FOR ANY ANAPHYLAXIS SYMPTOMS.

MUST BE COMPLETED BY HEALTHCARE PROVIDER, PARENT, AND SCHOOL NURSE

AUTHORIZATION

*Prescriber's Signature: _____ Date: _____
Printed Name: _____ Phone: _____
I confirm student is capable to safely carry and properly administer above medication ☐ Yes ☐ No

Parent/Guardian Consent: I have received, reviewed and understand the above information. I approve of this Allergy Action Plan. I give my permission for the school nurse and trained school personnel to follow this plan, administer medication(s), and contact my provider, if necessary. I assume full responsibility for providing the school with the prescribed medications. I give my permission for the school to share the above information with school staff that need to know about my child's condition.
ParentGuardian Signature: _____ Date: _____
I confirm my child is capable to safely carry and properly administer above medication ☐ Yes ☐ No

School Nurse
I have reviewed this order and completed the allergy emergency care plan and shared with trained school personnel.

Signature / Date _____

Medication Expires on: _____

Potential for altered respiratory status/anaphylaxis   Allergy Action Plan   Goal: Patent Airway

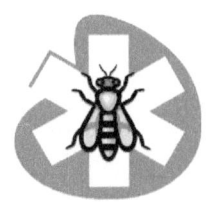

8. PROGRESS NOTES

Caregiver :

Patients Name :   Physicians Name :

Date	Note	Caregivers Initial

🐝 # PROGRESS NOTES

Patient Name

Weight	B.P	Blood Sugar	Other

Notes

Tuesday, March 24, 2015	Notes

PROGRESS NOTES

al Name	P/a Name	Attending Physician	Room No	Med. No
Date	Notes Should Be Signed by Physician			

🐝 **PROGRESS NOTES** ╱

Name_____

1st Session Chart

2nd Session Chart

Ryan Jay
Hoyme

PROGRESS NOTES

NAME _____ ID# _____

DATE	

PROGRESS NOTES

Name_____

1st Session Chart

2nd Session Chart

Ryan Jay
Hoyme

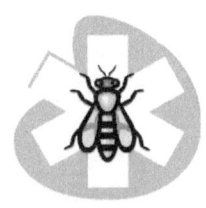

9. SOAP: SUBJECTIVE, OBJECTIVE, ASSESSMENT, PLAN

🐝   **SOAP NOTES**

Date of Therapy: **Patient/Client:**

Date of CURRENT: (Injury, Illness, or Pregnancy)

Attending Therapist: **Signature:**

S

O

A

P

SOAP NOTES

⚘

Client Name	
Date_____ Session #_____ S:_____ O:_____ A:_____ P:_____	Date_____ Session #_____ S:_____ O:_____ A:_____ P:_____
Date_____ Session #_____ S:_____ O:_____ A:_____ P:_____	Date_____ Session #_____ S:_____ O:_____ A:_____ P:_____
Date_____ Session #_____ S:_____ O:_____ A:_____ P:_____ Ryan Jay Hayne	Date_____ Session #_____ S:_____ O:_____ A:_____ P:_____

SOAP NOTES

		S	O	A	P				
Date	Prob. No. of Letter	Subjective	Objective	Assess	Plan				

SOAP NOTES

| No | Name | | DOB / / | TEST DONE CIRCLE OR TICK |

DATE | **WORKING DIAGNOSIS** | SAME ( ) | MILD MODERATE SEVERE | FLAGS | MUSCLE WEAKNESS. BLADDER/BOWEL GROIN NUMBNESS. SENSATION CHANGE | 1° 2° 3°

SUBJECTIVE COMPLAINT(S): AREAS: - NECK / DORSAL / LB / PELVIC / MAINT / OTHER -:

WORSE, SAME, EASIER, ALOT EASIER, VERY GOOD. (10 = SEVERE, 1= MILD) 0 1 2 3 4 5 6 7 8 9 10 N/A

PAIN FREQUENCY TRACE ≤ 10% OF DAY ≤ 20 ≤ 30 ≤ 40 ≤ 50 ≤ 60 ≤ 70 ≤ 80 ≤ 90 ≤ 100% ZERO

PERCENTAGE PROBLEM IMPROVED WITH TREATMENT: 0% 10% 20% 30% 40% 50% 60% 70% 80% 90% 100% N/A

OBJECTIVE FINDINGS: MOVEMENT/ LOCOMOTION: NORM, GUARDED, ABNOR, RESTRICTED, OTHER:

PALPATION /OBSERVATION: TENDERNESS. M.SPASM. NUMBNESS. SWELLING. FIXATION, HYPERMOBILITY, ATROPHY. OK

ASSESSMENT / TESTS / RX: SLR (L)(R), SLUMP (L)(R), TOE EXTENSORS (L)(R), S1 REFLEX (L)(R).

O = STIFF X = PAINFUL OO = V. STIFF XX = V. PAINFUL R

FIXATIONS: Occ C1 C2 C3 C4 C5 C6 C7 T1 T2 T3 T4 T5 T6 T7 T8 T9 T10 T11 T12 L1 L2 L3 L4 L5 Sac Coc

S/T THERAPY - ( ) MASSAGER - ( ). FASCIAL RELEASE - ( )
INTERFERENTIAL - ( ). ULTRASOUND ( ). MOBILISATION - ( )

| | POST TREATMENT | NEXT APPOINTMENT | SIGNED |

PLAN: ICE, REST, HEAT, SHORT WALKS, DIET, SUPPORT, POSTURAL ADVICE, ADVICE AT WORK, TAPING, NSAIDS, PARACETAMOL, EXERCISES - ( )

DATE | **WORKING DIAGNOSIS** | SAME ( ) | MILD MODERATE SEVERE | FLAGS | MUSCLE WEAKNESS. BLADDER/BOWEL GROIN NUMBNESS. SENSATION CHANGE | 1° 2° 3°

SUBJECTIVE COMPLAINT(S): AREAS: - NECK / DORSAL / LB / PELVIC / MAINT / OTHER -:

WORSE, SAME, EASIER, ALOT EASIER, VERY GOOD. (10 = SEVERE, 1= MILD) 0 1 2 3 4 5 6 7 8 9 10 N/A

PAIN FREQUENCY TRACE ≤ 10% OF DAY ≤ 20 ≤ 30 ≤ 40 ≤ 50 ≤ 60 ≤ 70 ≤ 80 ≤ 90 ≤ 100% ZERO

PERCENTAGE PROBLEM IMPROVED WITH TREATMENT: 0% 10% 20% 30% 40% 50% 60% 70% 80% 90% 100% N/A

OBJECTIVE FINDINGS: MOVEMENT/ LOCOMOTION: NORM, GUARDED, ABNOR, RESTRICTED, OTHER:

PALPATION /OBSERVATION: TENDERNESS. M.SPASM. NUMBNESS. SWELLING. FIXATION, HYPERMOBILITY, ATROPHY. OK

ASSESSMENT / TESTS / RX: SLR (L)(R), SLUMP (L)(R), TOE EXTENSORS (L)(R), S1 REFLEX (L)(R).

O = STIFF X = PAINFUL OO = V. STIFF XX = V. PAINFUL R

FIXATIONS: Occ C1 C2 C3 C4 C5 C6 C7 T1 T2 T3 T4 T5 T6 T7 T8 T9 T10 T11 T12 L1 L2 L3 L4 L5 Sac Coc

S/T THERAPY - ( ) MASSAGER - ( ). FASCIAL RELEASE - ( )
INTERFERENTIAL - ( ). ULTRASOUND ( ). MOBILISATION - ( )

| | POST TREATMENT | NEXT APPOINTMENT | SIGNED |

PLAN: ICE, REST, HEAT, SHORT WALKS, DIET, SUPPORT, POSTURAL ADVICE, ADVICE AT WORK, TAPING, NSAIDS, PARACETAMOL, EXERCISES - ( )

DATE | **WORKING DIAGNOSIS** | SAME ( ) | MILD MODERATE SEVERE | FLAGS | MUSCLE WEAKNESS. BLADDER/BOWEL GROIN NUMBNESS. SENSATION CHANGE | 1° 2° 3°

SUBJECTIVE COMPLAINT(S): AREAS: - NECK / DORSAL / LB / PELVIC / MAINT / OTHER -:

WORSE, SAME, EASIER, ALOT EASIER, VERY GOOD. (10 = SEVERE, 1= MILD) 0 1 2 3 4 5 6 7 8 9 10 N/A

PAIN FREQUENCY TRACE ≤ 10% OF DAY ≤ 20 ≤ 30 ≤ 40 ≤ 50 ≤ 60 ≤ 70 ≤ 80 ≤ 90 ≤ 100% ZERO

PERCENTAGE PROBLEM IMPROVED WITH TREATMENT: 0% 10% 20% 30% 40% 50% 60% 70% 80% 90% 100% N/A

OBJECTIVE FINDINGS: MOVEMENT/LOCOMOTION: NORM, GUARDED, ABNOR, RESTRICTED, OTHER:

PALPATION /OBSERVATION: TENDERNESS. M.SPASM. NUMBNESS. SWELLING. FIXATION, HYPERMOBILITY, ATROPHY. OK

ASSESSMENT / TESTS / RX: SLR (L)(R), SLUMP (L)(R), TOE EXTENSORS (L)(R), S1 REFLEX (L)(R).

O = STIFF X = PAINFUL OO = V. STIFF XX = V. PAINFUL R

FIXATIONS: Occ C1 C2 C3 C4 C5 C6 C7 T1 T2 T3 T4 T5 T6 T7 T8 T9 T10 T11 T12 L1 L2 L3 L4 L5 Sac Coc

S/T THERAPY - ( ) MASSAGER - ( ). FASCIAL RELEASE - ( )
INTERFERENTIAL - ( ). ULTRASOUND ( ). MOBILISATION - ( )

| | POST TREATMENT | NEXT APPOINTMENT | SIGNED |

PLAN: ICE, REST, HEAT, SHORT WALKS, DIET, SUPPORT, POSTURAL ADVICE, ADVICE AT WORK, TAPING, NSAIDS, PARACETAMOL, EXERCISES - ( )

NOTES

SOAP NOTES

Patient
Name:_____

Date:_____ Age:_____ Sex:_____

SUBJECTIVE: (Mechanism of injury (MOI), chief complaint (C/C))
_____
_____
_____
_____
_____

OBJECTIVE: (Patient exam findings, Vital Signs, SAMPLE History)
Vital Signs:

Time:				
LOC:				
HR				
RR				
Skin (C/T/M)				

Patient Exam: Describe locations of pain, tenderness, injuries, Pertinent negatives
_____
_____
_____
_____
_____

SAMPLE:
Signs/Symptoms:
Allergies:
Medications:
Pertinent Medical History:
Last Oral Intake:
Events leading to accident:

ASSESSMENT: (problem list)
1._____
2._____
3._____
4._____
5._____

PLAN: (plan for each problem on list, evac route, bivouac location)
1._____
2._____
3._____
4._____
5._____

SOAP NOTES

COMPANY: _____

DOCTOR: _____

DATE: __/__/__

Name: Primary:
PAN: Secondary:
Date: Record:

Diagnosis   **Procedures**

Subjective:

Objective:

Assessment:

Plan:

SOAP NOTES

Client Name_____

Date_____
Session #_____
S:_____

O:_____
_____

A:_____

P:_____
_____
_____

Date_____
Session #_____
S:_____

O:_____
_____

A:_____

P:_____
_____

Date_____
Session #_____
S:_____

O:_____
_____

A:_____

P:_____
_____
_____

Date_____
Session #_____
S:_____

O:_____
_____

A:_____

P:_____
_____

Date_____
Session #_____
S:_____

O:_____

A:_____

P:_____
_____

Ryan Jay Hoyne

Date_____
Session #_____
S:_____

O:_____

A:_____

P:_____
_____

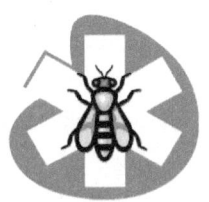

10. MEASURES AND CONVERSIONS

POSOLOGY: APPROXIMATE CONVERSIONS IN VOLUME AND WEIGHT

BEE VENOM (APITOXIN)

- 1 bee sting = 0.1 mg dry venom
- 1 mg dry venom = 10 bee stings
- 1 g dry venom = 10,000 bee stings
- Lethal dose = @ 600 bee stings (in an adult)
- Potential risk of anaphylactic shock = 1/150,500

HONEY
- 1 teaspoon = 8,0 g = 5 mL = 22 calories
- 1 tablespoon (3 teasp.) = 24.0 g = 1.0 ounce = 15 mL = 64 cal
- 1 cup (16 tablespoons) = 384.0 g = 250 mL = 1031 calories

POLLEN
- 1 level teaspoon = 5.0 g
- 1 heaping teaspoon = 8.0 g
- 1 level dessertspoon = 10.0 g
- 1 heaping dessertspoon = 15.0 g
- 1 level spoon = 15.0 g
- 1 heaping spoon = 24.0 g
- 1 tablespoon = 3 teaspoons = 1.5 dessertspoon

PROPOLIS TINCTURE OR EXTRACT
- 1 drop = 0.05 mL
- 1 dropper (20 drops) = 1.0 mL
- 1 dropper of 30 % tincture = 0.3 g of pure propolis
- 1 teaspoon = 5.0 mL
- 1 tablespoon = 15.0 mL
- 1 cup = 240 mL

ROYAL JELLY
- 1 teaspoon = 5500 mg

VITAMIN INTERNATIONAL UNITS
- 1000 IU vitamin A = 600 µg β-carotene
- 1000 IU vitamin C = 50 mg L-ascorbic acid
- 1000 IU vitamin D = 25 µg cholecalciferol
- 1000 IU vitamin E = 667 mg d-α-tocopherol acetate

POSOLOGÍA: EQUIVALENTES APROXIMADOS EN VOLUMEN Y PESO

JALEA REAL
- 1 cucharadita (cdta.) de café = 5500 mg

MIEL
- 1 cucharadita de café = 8,0 g = 5 mL = 22 calorías
- 1 cucharada (3 cdtas.) = 24,0 g = 1,0 onza = 15 mL = 64 calorías
- 1 taza (16 cucharadas) = 384,0 g = 250 mL = 1031 calorías

POLEN
- 1 cucharadita de café rasa = 5,0 g
- 1 cucharadita de café colmada = 8,0 g
- 1 cucharadita de postre rasa = 10,0 g
- 1 cucharadita de postre colmada = 15,0 g
- 1 cucharada rasa = 15,0 g
- 1 cucharada colmada = 24,0 g
- 1 cucharada = 3 cucharaditas de café = 1,5 cdta. de postre

PROPÓLEO TINTURA O EXTRACTO
- 1 gota = 0,05 mL
- 1 gotero (20 gotas) = 1,0 mL
- 1 gotero de tintura al 30 % = 0,3 g de propóleo puro
- 1 cucharadita = 5,0 mL
- 1 cucharada = 15,0 mL
- 1 taza = 240 mL

VENENO DE ABEJAS (APITOXINA)
- 1 picadura de abeja = 0,1 mg de veneno seco
- 1 mg de veneno seco = 10 picaduras
- 1 g de veneno seco = 10 000 picaduras
- Dosis letal = @ 600 picaduras (en un adulto)
- Riesgo potencial de reacción anafiláctica = 1/150 500

UNIDADES INTERNACIONALES DE VITAMINAS
- 1000 UI de vitamina A = 600 µg de β-caroteno
- 1000 UI de vitamina C = 50 mg de ácido L-ascórbico
- 1000 UI de vitamina D = 25 µg de colecalciferol
- 1000 UI de vitamina E = 667 mg de acetato de d-α-tocoferol

VOLUME CONVERSIONS

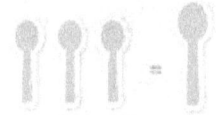

3 tsp. = 1 tbsp.

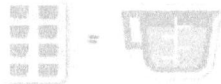

8 fluid oz. = 1 cup

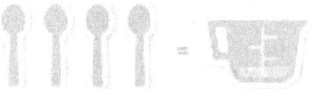

4 tbsp. = 1/4 cup.

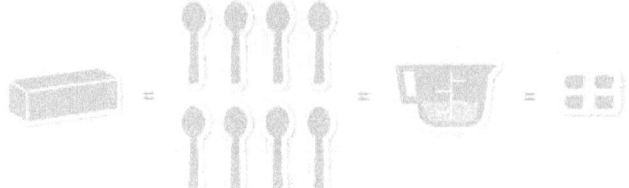

1 stick butter = 8 tbsp. = 1/2 cup = 4 oz.

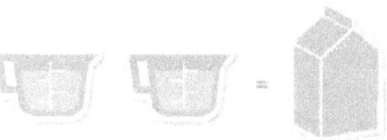

2 cups = 1 pint

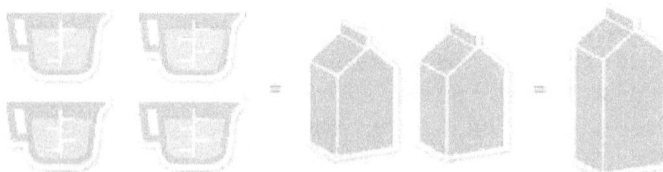

4 cups = 2 pints = 1 quart

Conversiones en volumen

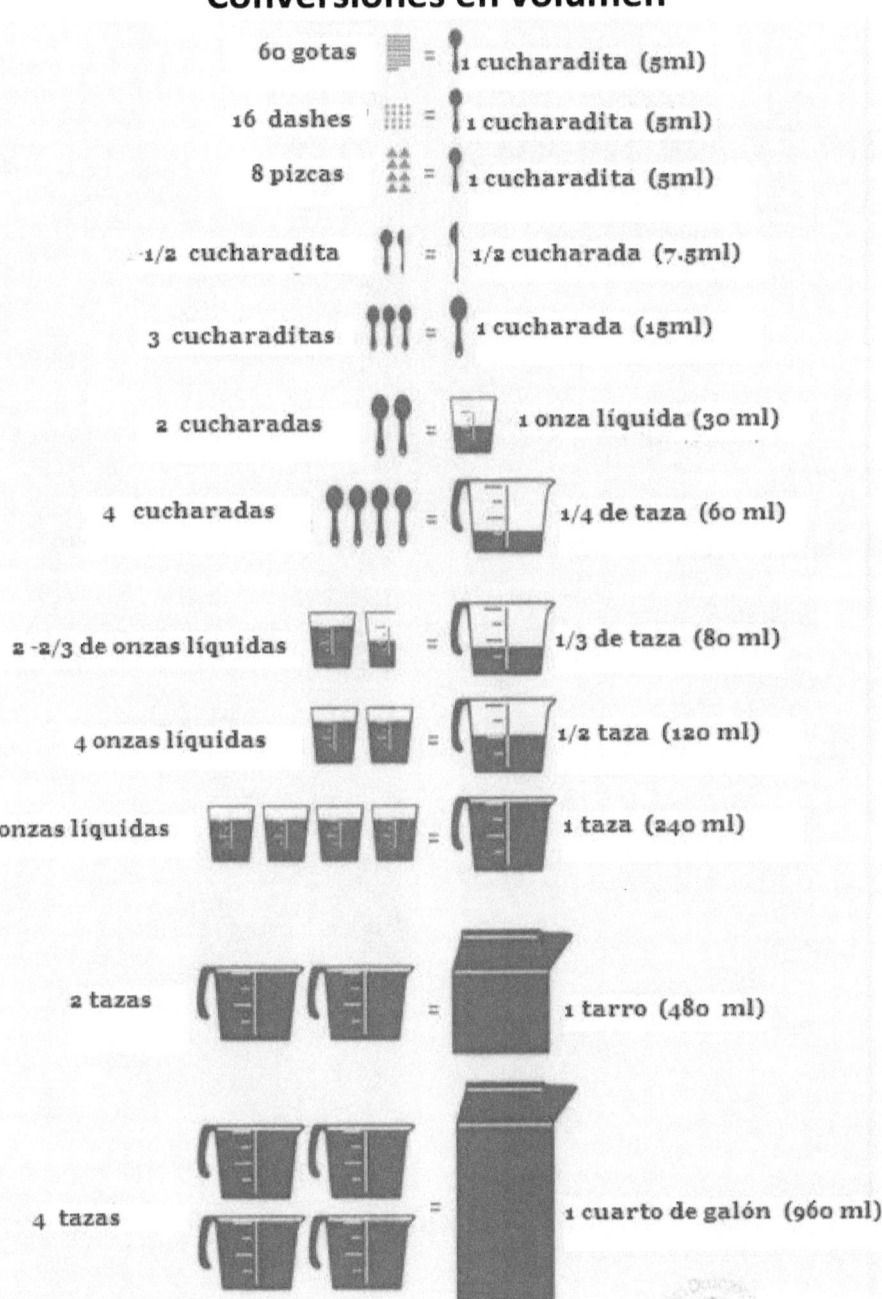

60 gotas = 1 cucharadita (5ml)

16 dashes = 1 cucharadita (5ml)

8 pizcas = 1 cucharadita (5ml)

1/2 cucharadita = 1/2 cucharada (7.5ml)

3 cucharaditas = 1 cucharada (15ml)

2 cucharadas = 1 onza líquida (30 ml)

4 cucharadas = 1/4 de taza (60 ml)

2 -2/3 de onzas líquidas = 1/3 de taza (80 ml)

4 onzas líquidas = 1/2 taza (120 ml)

8 onzas líquidas = 1 taza (240 ml)

2 tazas = 1 tarro (480 ml)

4 tazas = 1 cuarto de galón (960 ml)

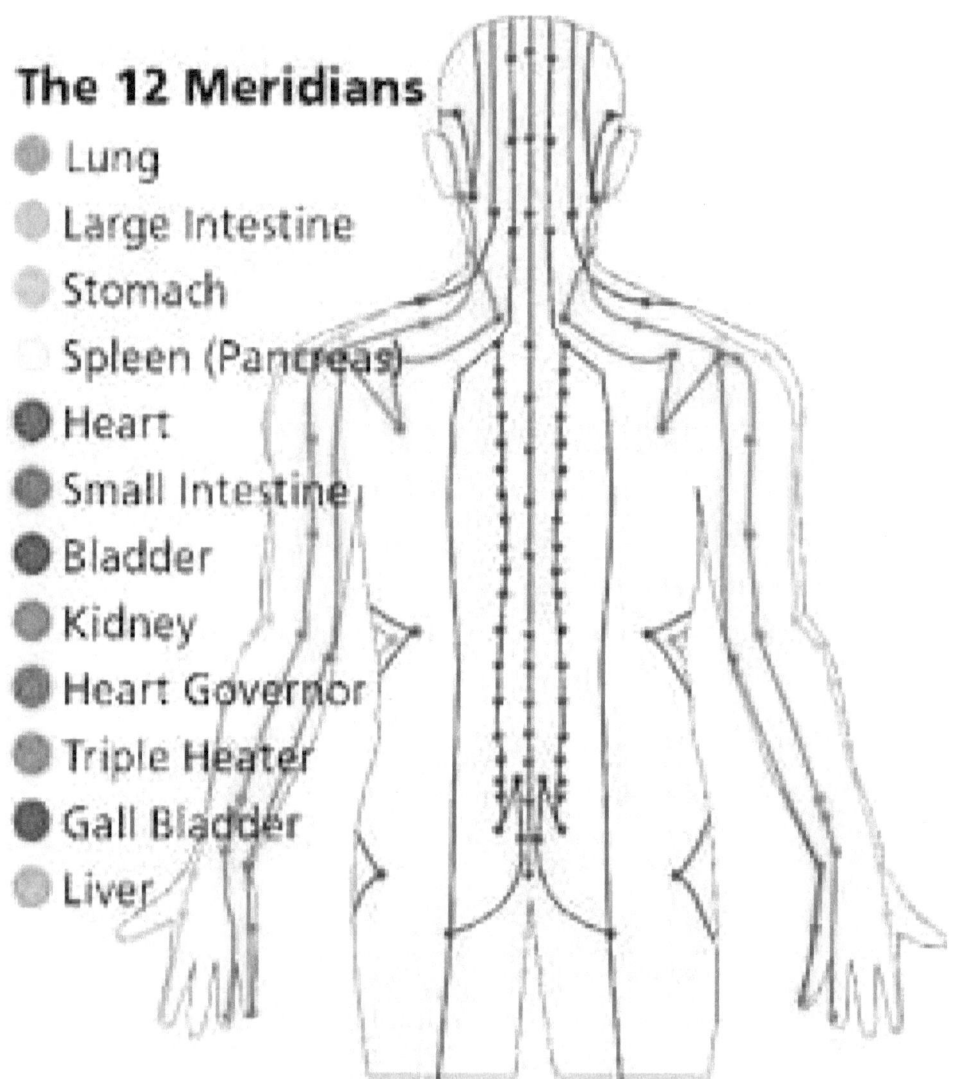

The 12 Meridians
- Lung
- Large Intestine
- Stomach
- Spleen (Pancreas)
- Heart
- Small Intestine
- Bladder
- Kidney
- Heart Governor
- Triple Heater
- Gall Bladder
- Liver

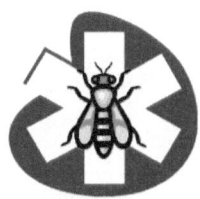

11.   MERIDIANS FOR APIPUNCTURE

Acupuncture points are used not only for treating disorders by stimulating or inhibiting those energy meridians with needles and moxas, but apitherapists also use those points for applying bee stings, micro-stings, and stipers and massages with honey, bee venom, propolis, and other bee products.

Diagrams are presented in two versions for each meridian. Meridians and points are identified in diagrams in English and in Spanish with their corresponding abbreviations. A much-extended practice is to use Spanish abbreviations for designating acupuncture points, but also English is preferred by many practitioners. It is better if you make copies of the following apipuncture diagrams and use them for your clients.

Once you have selected all the pertinent apipuncture meridians and points for a client, according to the diagnosis, circle with a color marker the selected points on the paper copy and this will make easier to mark in color the selected points on the skin for applying bee stings, bee venom injections, micro-stings, stipers, or massage.

Two meridians are axial, six meridians of arms are *yin*, and six meridians of legs are *yang*. Each meridian is related to a set of organs and body functions. Other classifications mention 12 regular meridians, 8 extraordinary meridians, and 15 bilateral meridians. In total, there are more than 7000 acupuncture points, also used in apipuncture.

Axial or extraordinary meridians:

- Conception vessel (CV), *yin* meridian: 24 axial points.
- Governing vessel (GV), *yang* meridian: 28 axial points.

Yin meridians or channels of arms:
- Heart (HT): 9 bilateral points.
- Pericardium (PC): 9 bilateral points.
- Lung (LU): 11 bilateral points.

Yin meridians or channels of legs:
- Spleen (SP): 21 bilateral points.
- Liver (LV): 14 bilateral points.
- Kidney (KI): 27 bilateral points.

Yang meridians or channels of arms:
- Small intestine (SI): 19 bilateral points.
- Large intestine (LI): 20 bilateral points.
- Triple heater (TH): 23 bilateral points.

Yang meridians or channels of legs:
- Stomach (ST): 45 bilateral points.
- Urinary bladder (UB): 67 bilateral points.
- Gall bladder (GB): 44 bilateral points.

☞   CV: CONCEPTION VESSEL

Name:

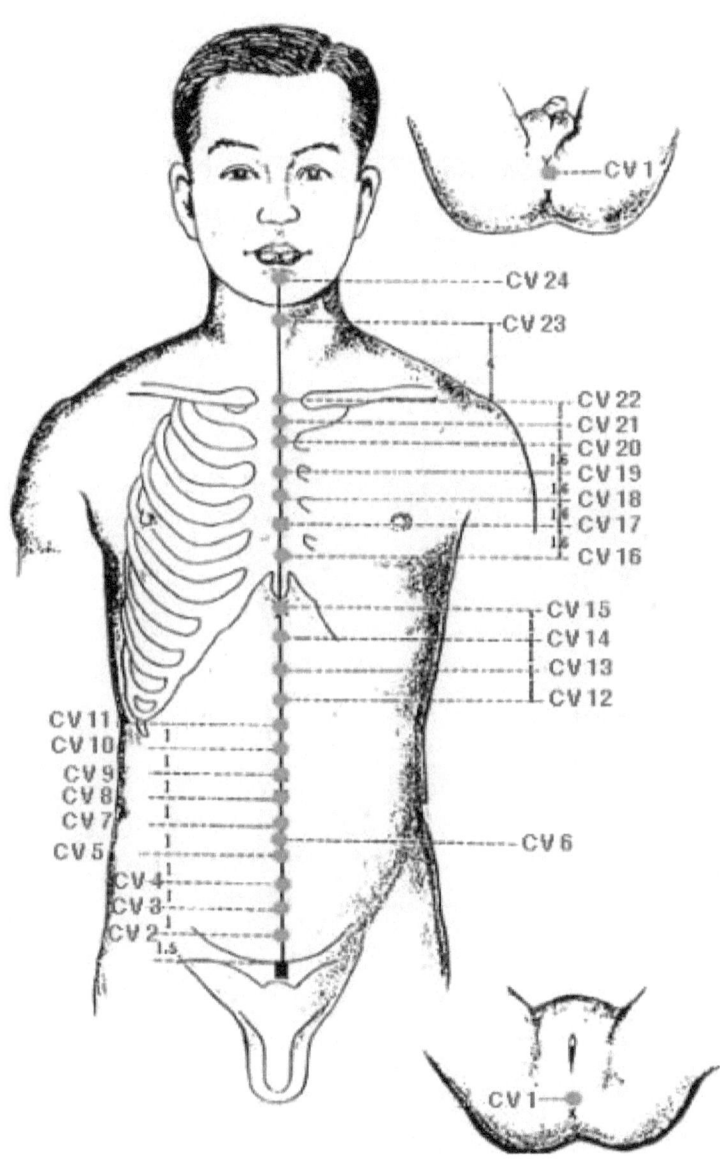

⚜ VC: Vaso concepción
Nombre:

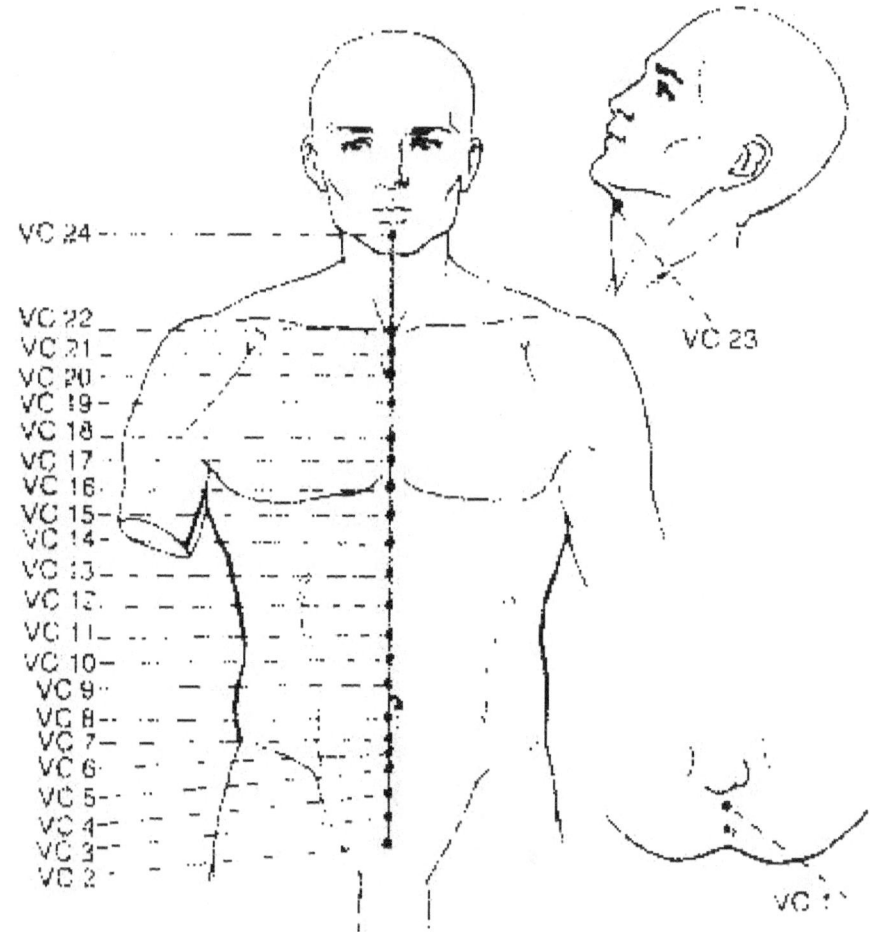

🐝 **GV: GOVERNING VESSEL**

Name:

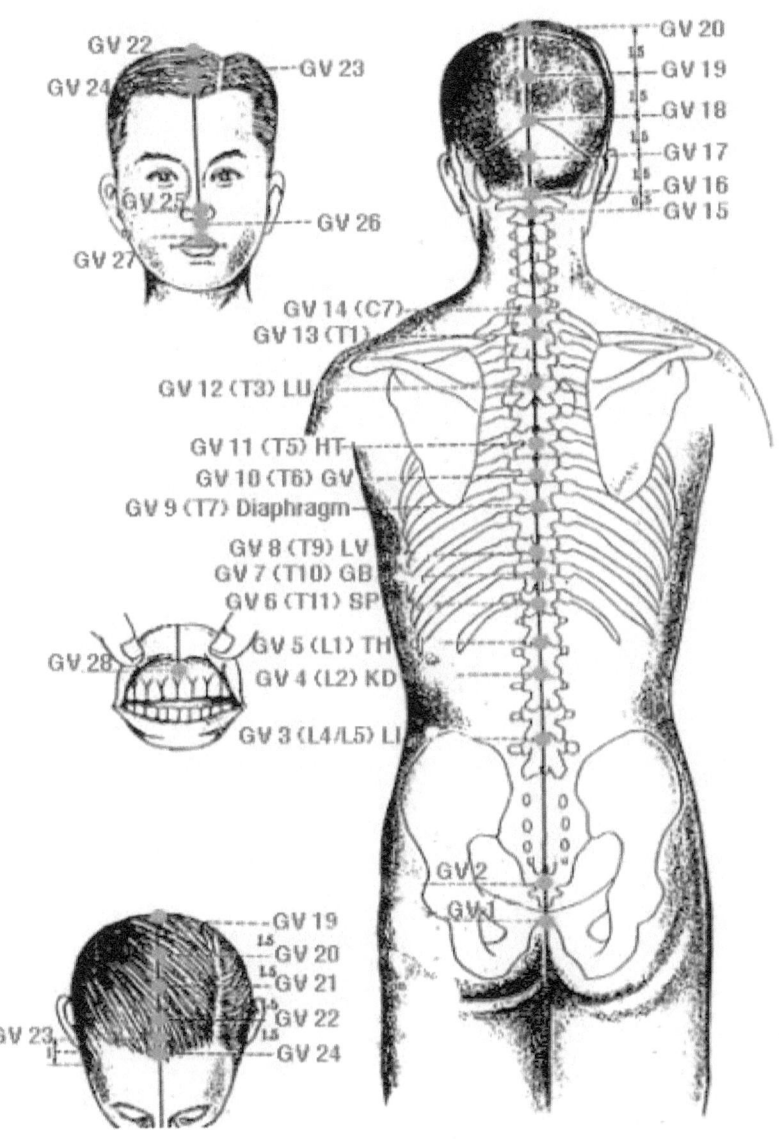

☞ VG: Vaso gobernador

Nombre:

☃ **HT: HEART**

Name:

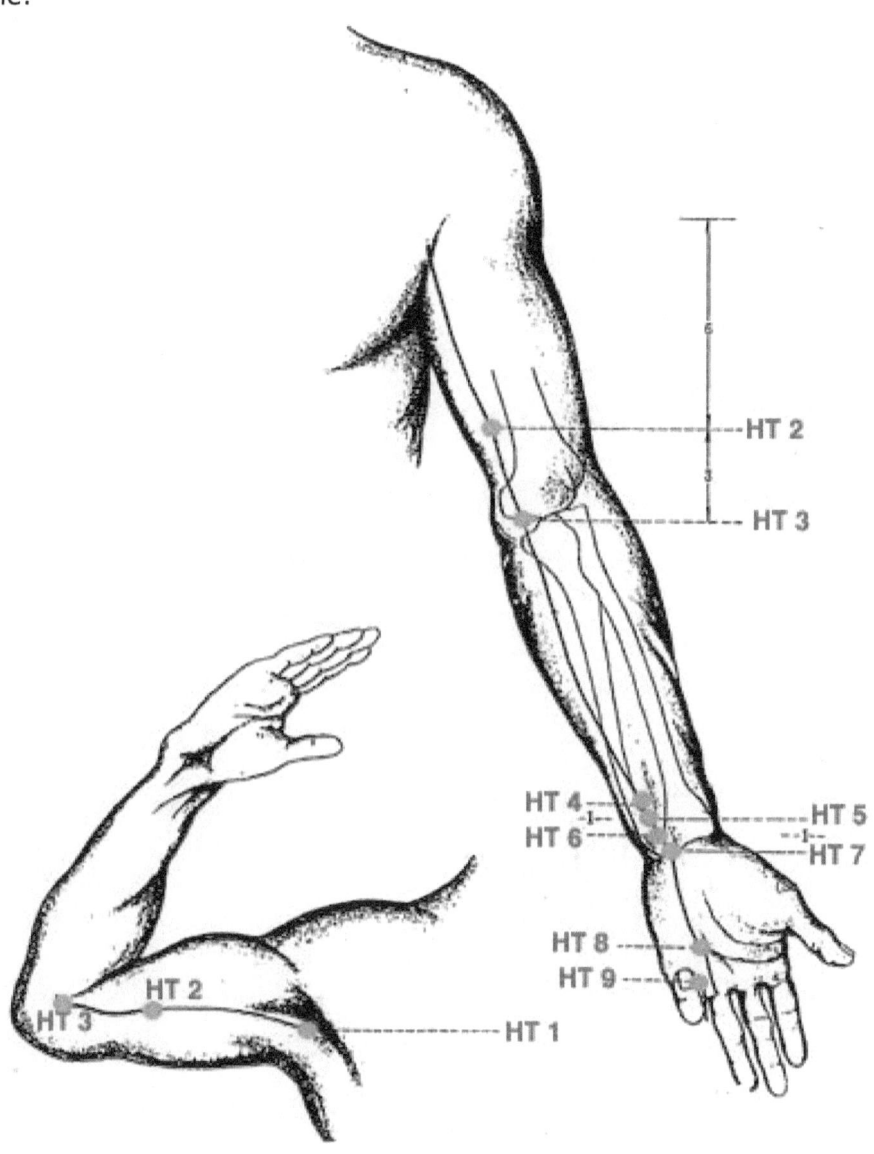

🐝 **C: Corazón**

Nombre:

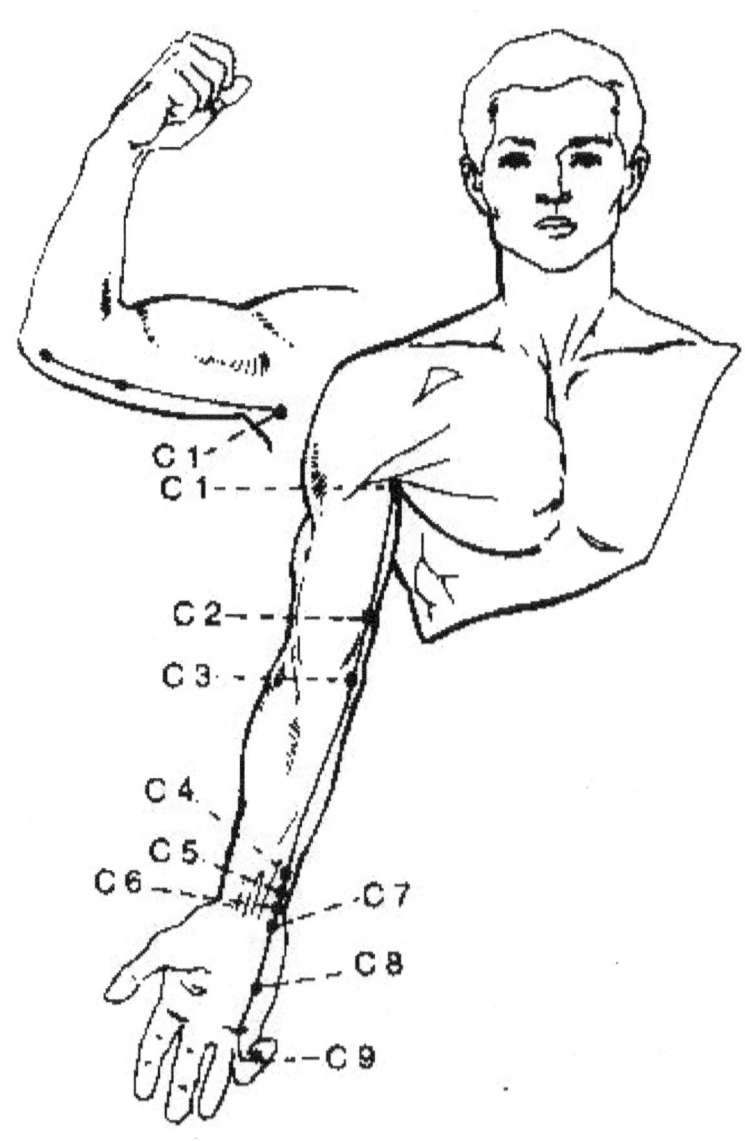

⊛ PC: PERICARDIUM

Name:

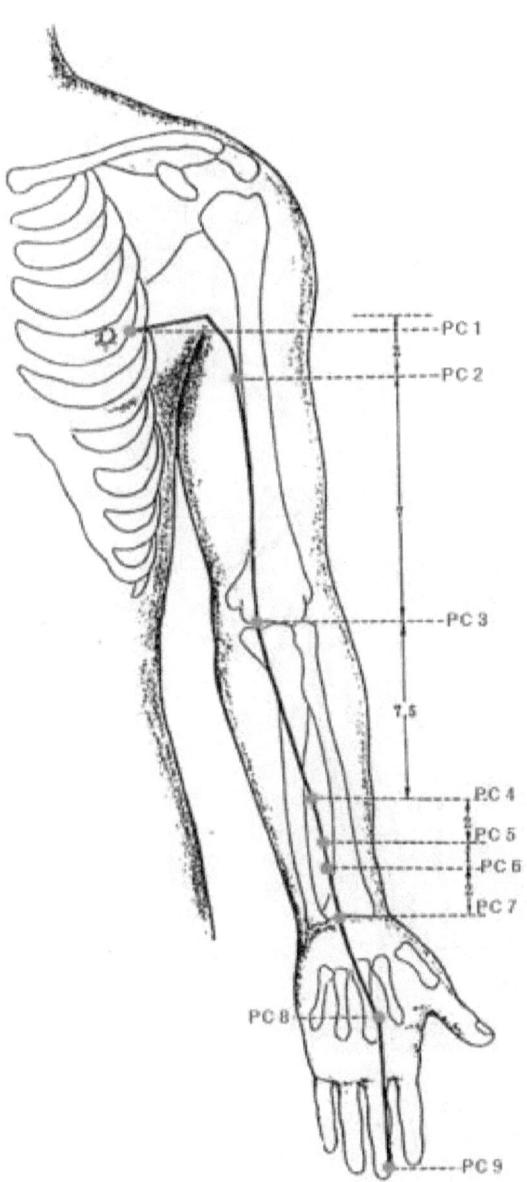

⚘   CS: Circulación-Sexualidad

Nombre:

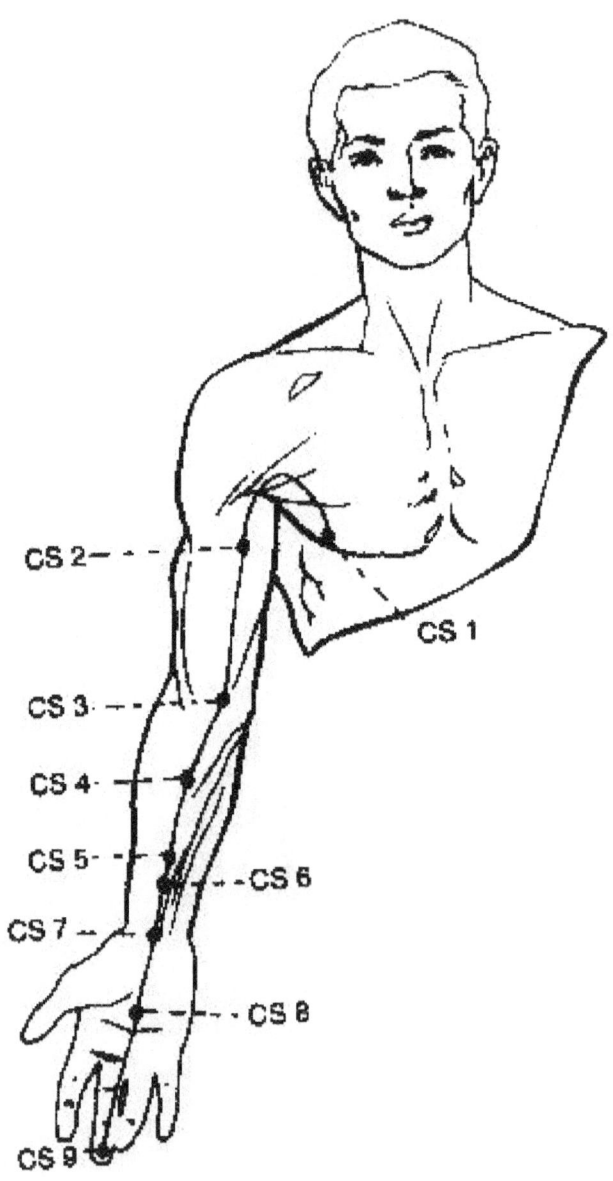

⊛ LU: LUNG

Name:

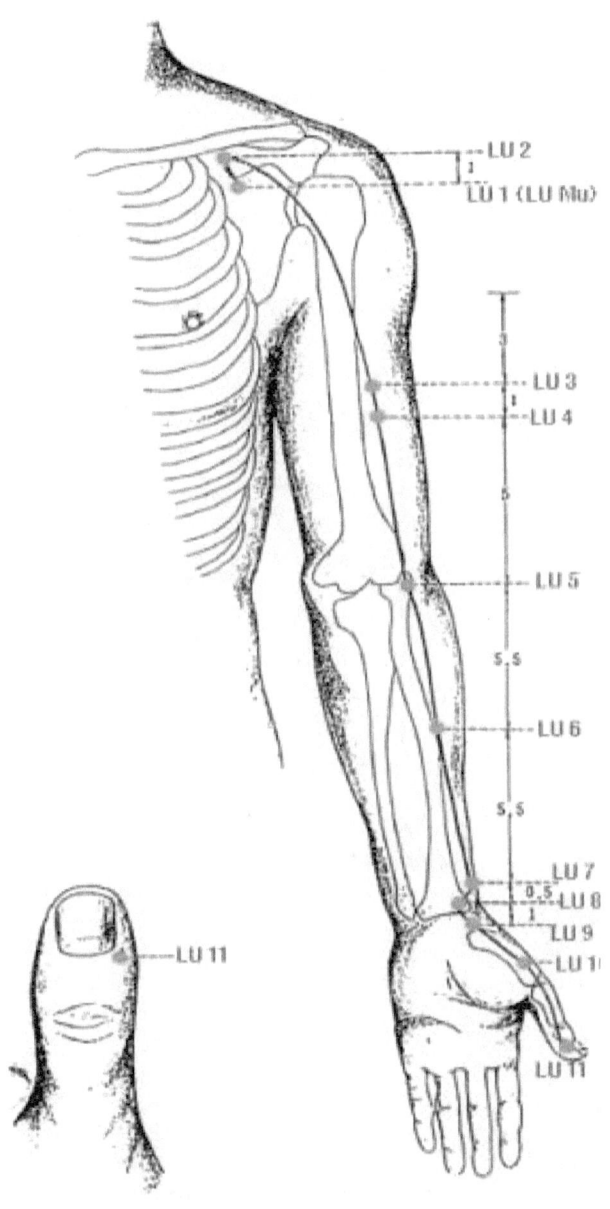

⊛ **P: Pulmón**

Nombre:

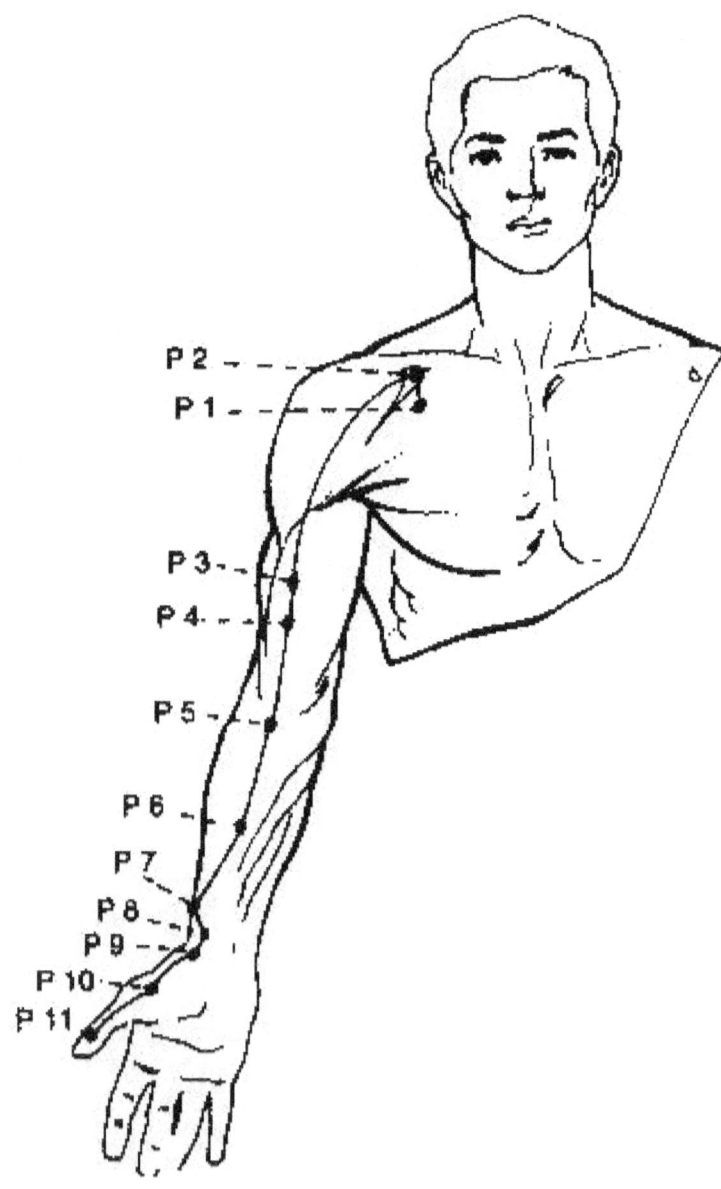

⑧ **SP: SPLEEN**

Name:

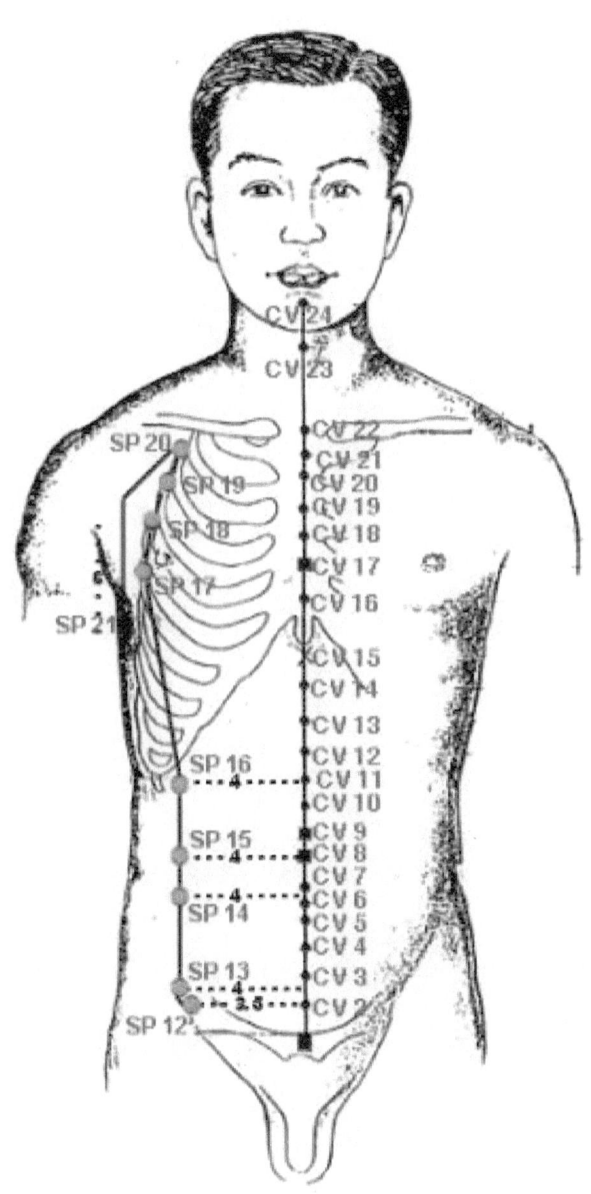

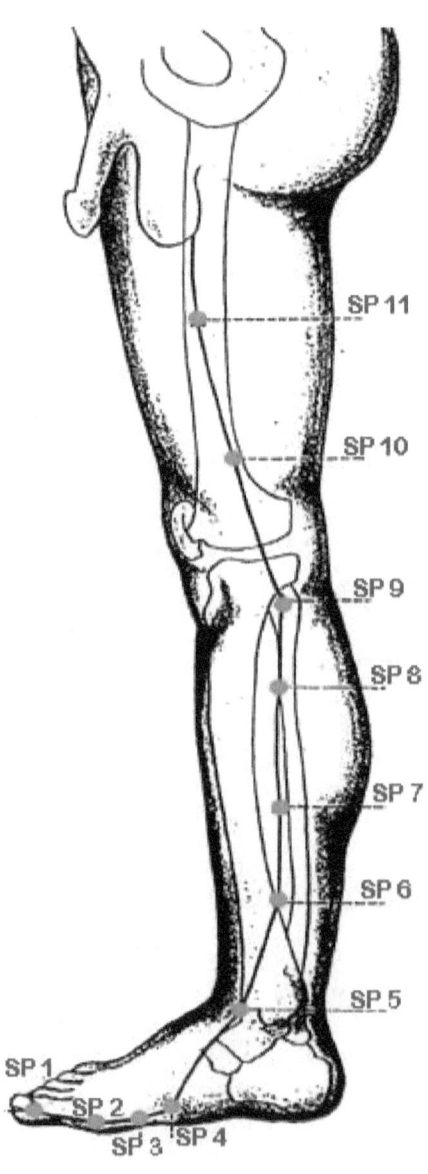

🐝 BP: Bazo-páncreas

Nombre:

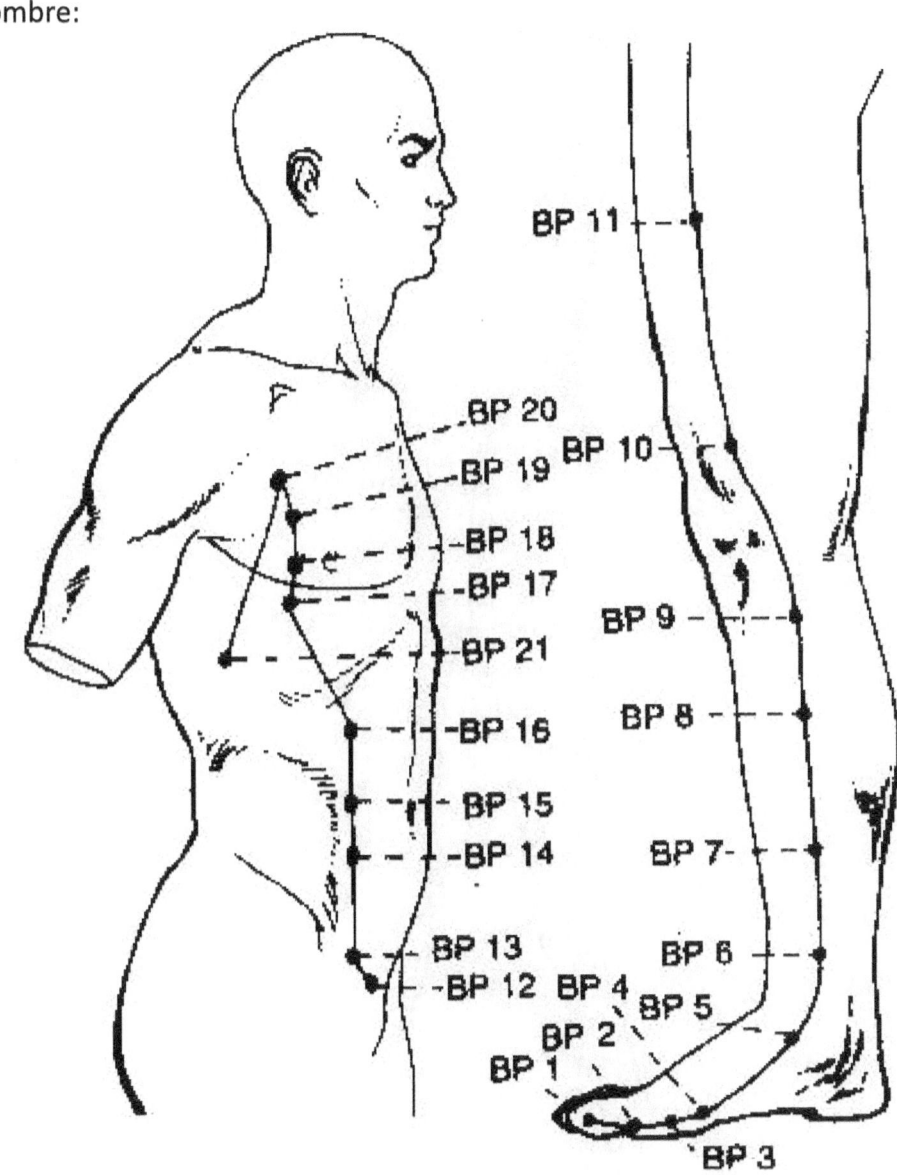

❊ LV: LIVER

Name:

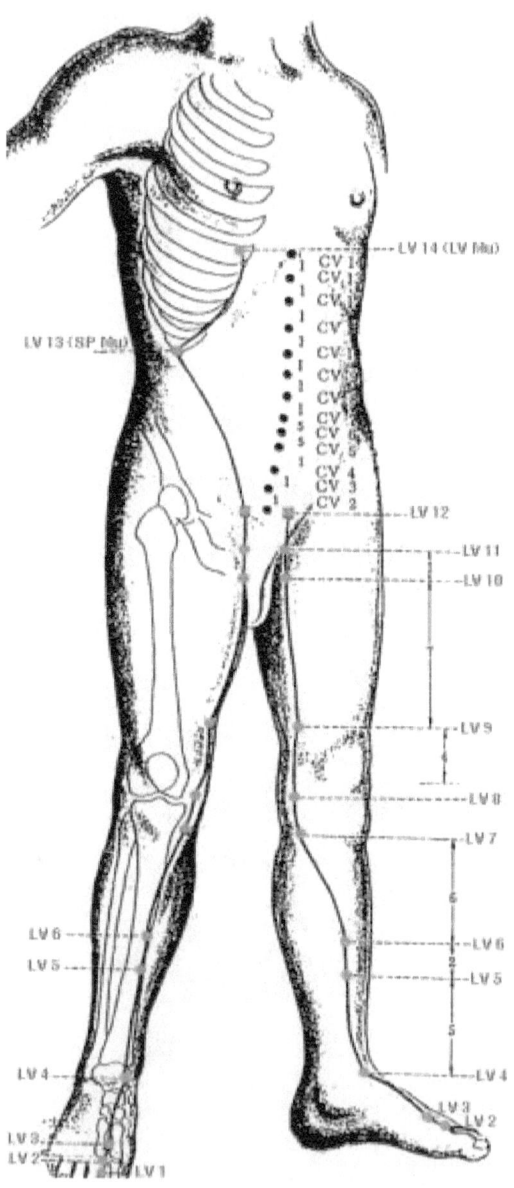

⊛ **H: Hígado**

Nombre:

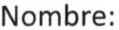

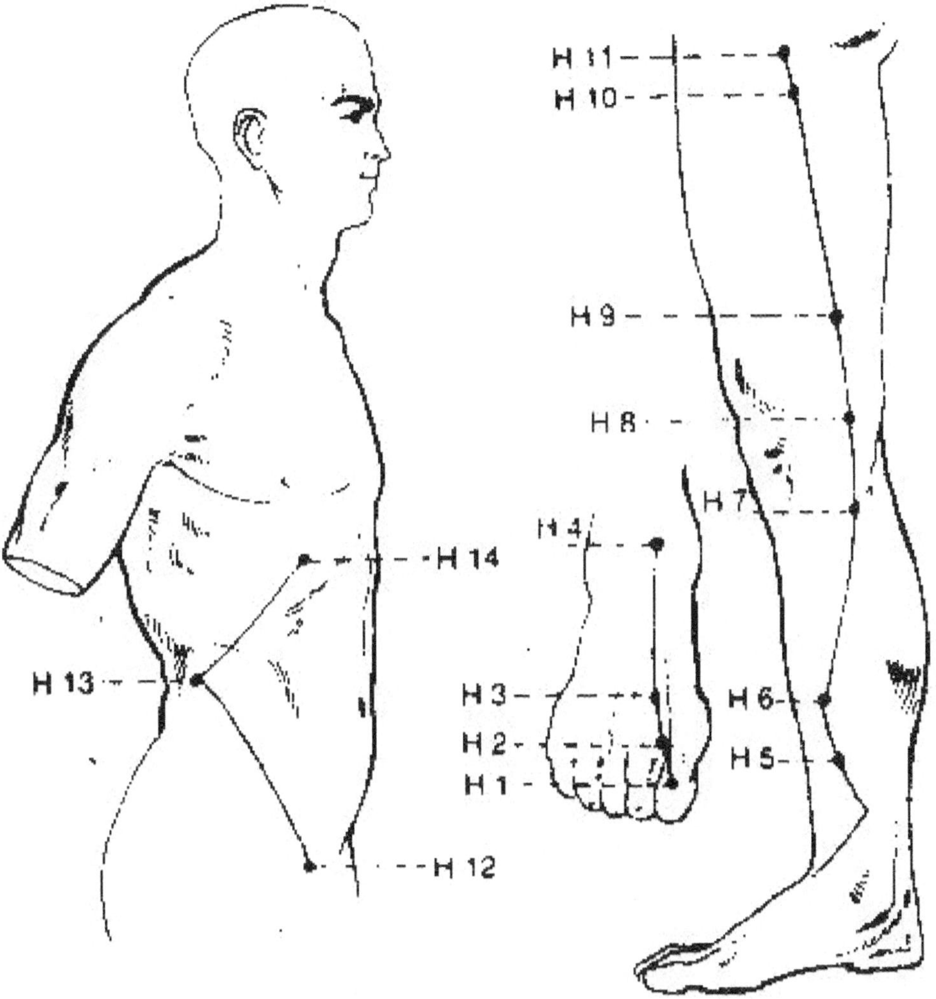

⊛ KD: KIDNEY

Name:

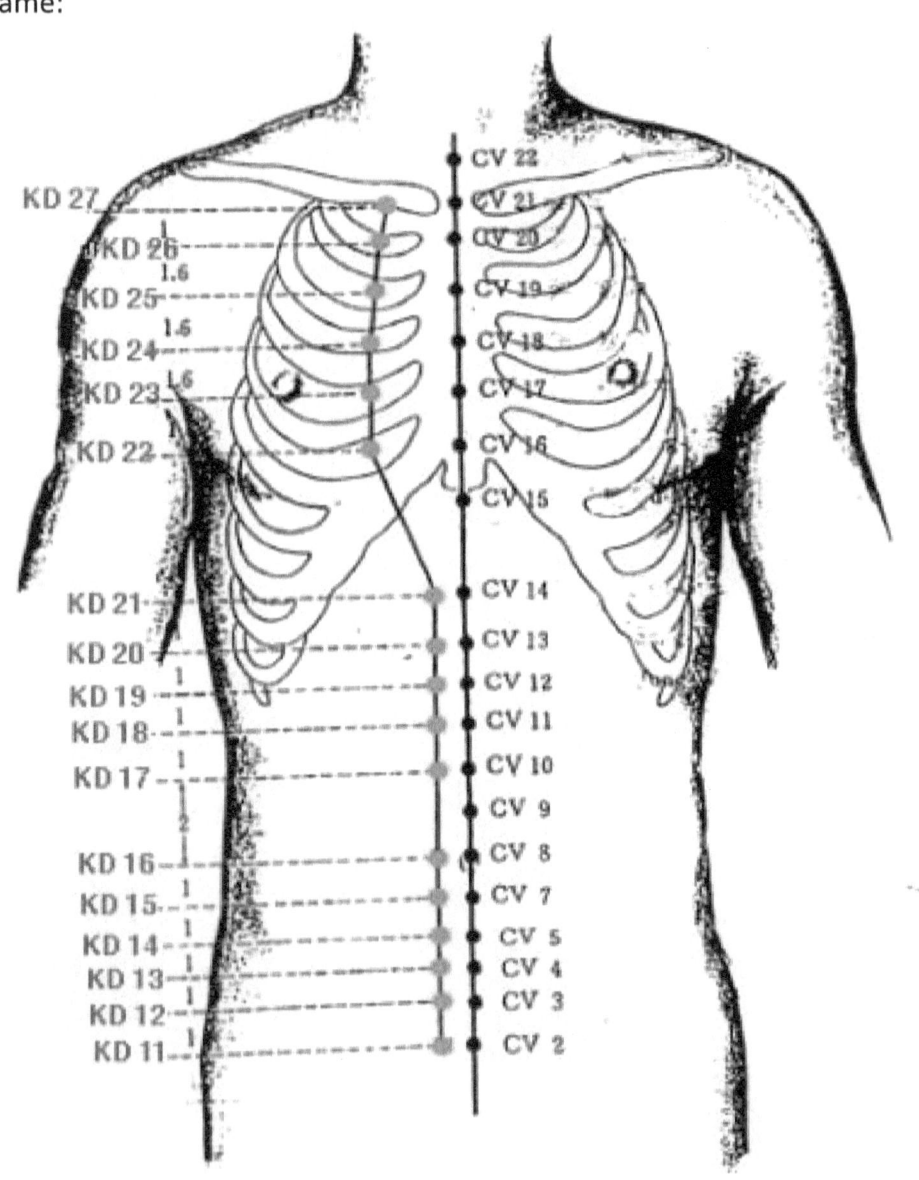

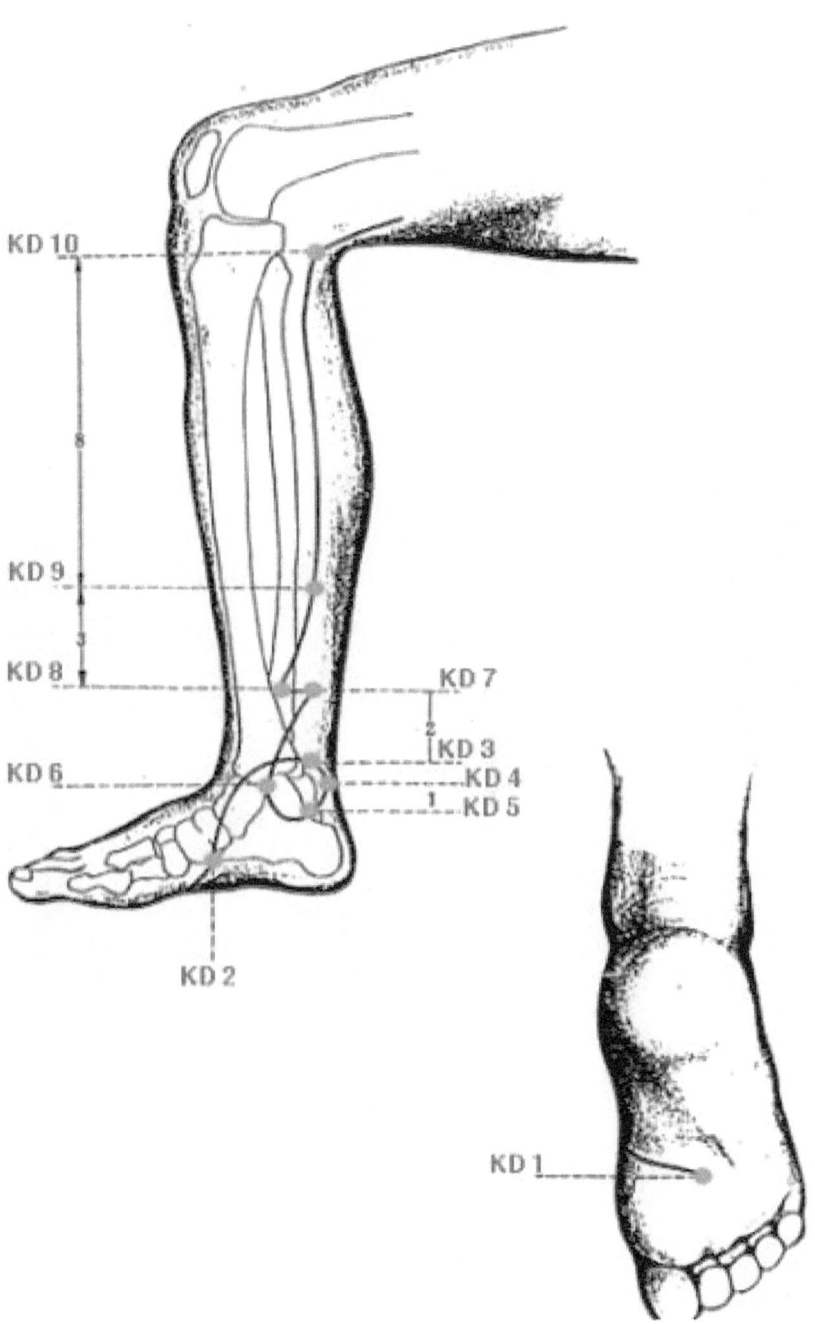

⊛ **R: Riñón**

Nombre:

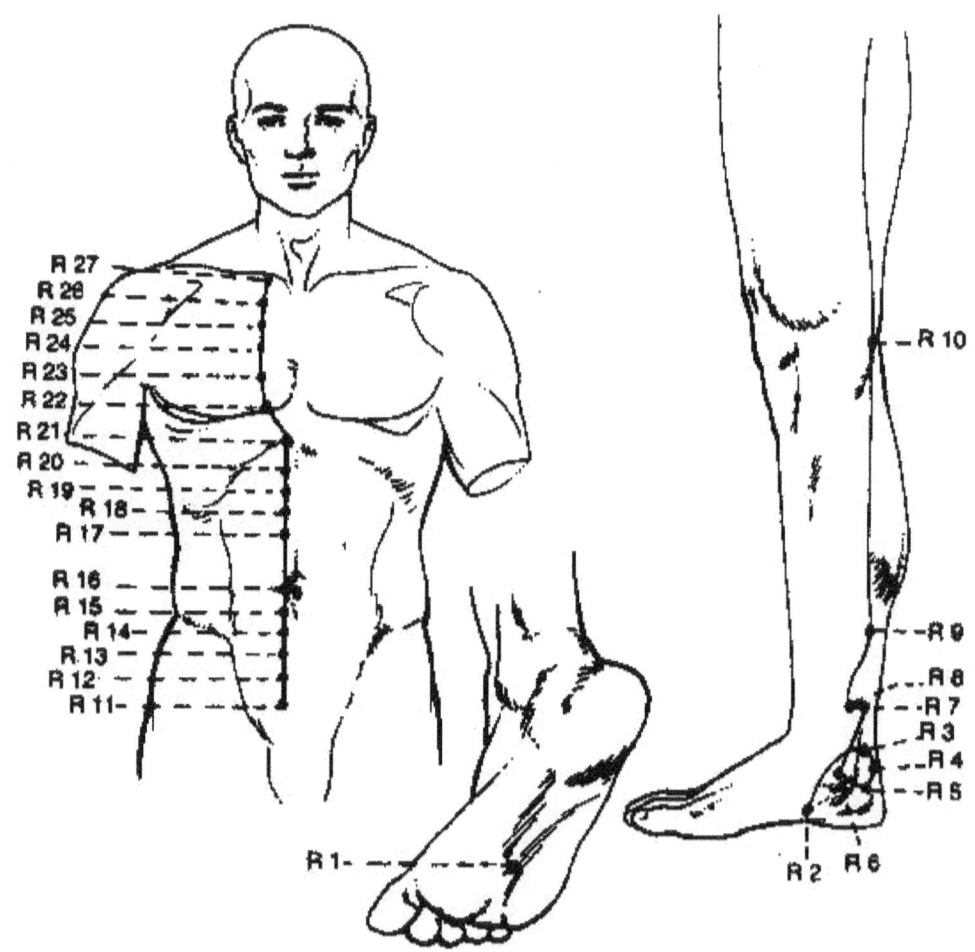

☖ SI: SMALL INTESTINE:

Name:

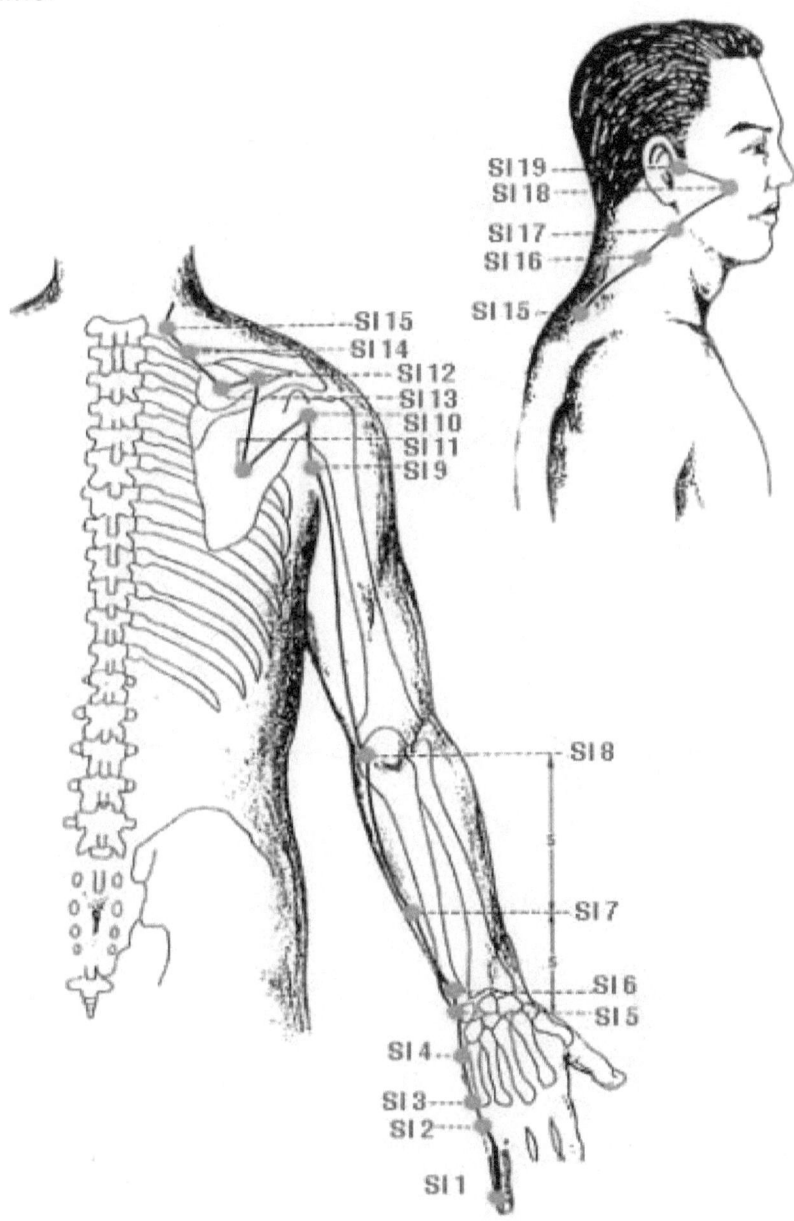

☸ ID: Intestino delgado
Nombre:

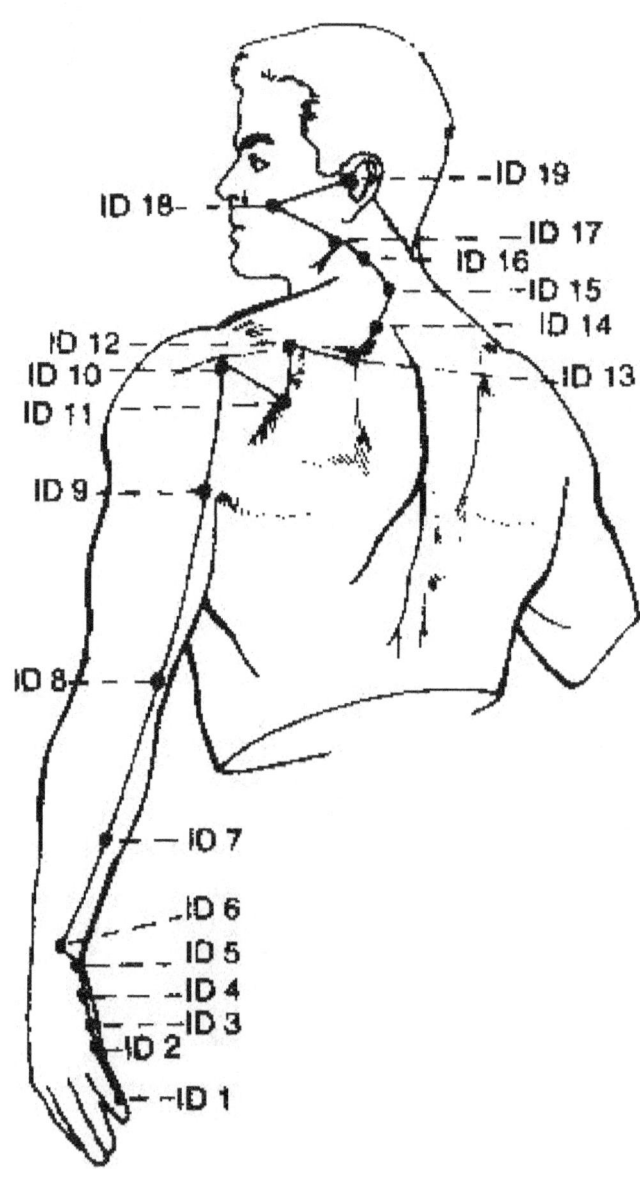

⊛ LI: LARGE INTESTINE

Name:

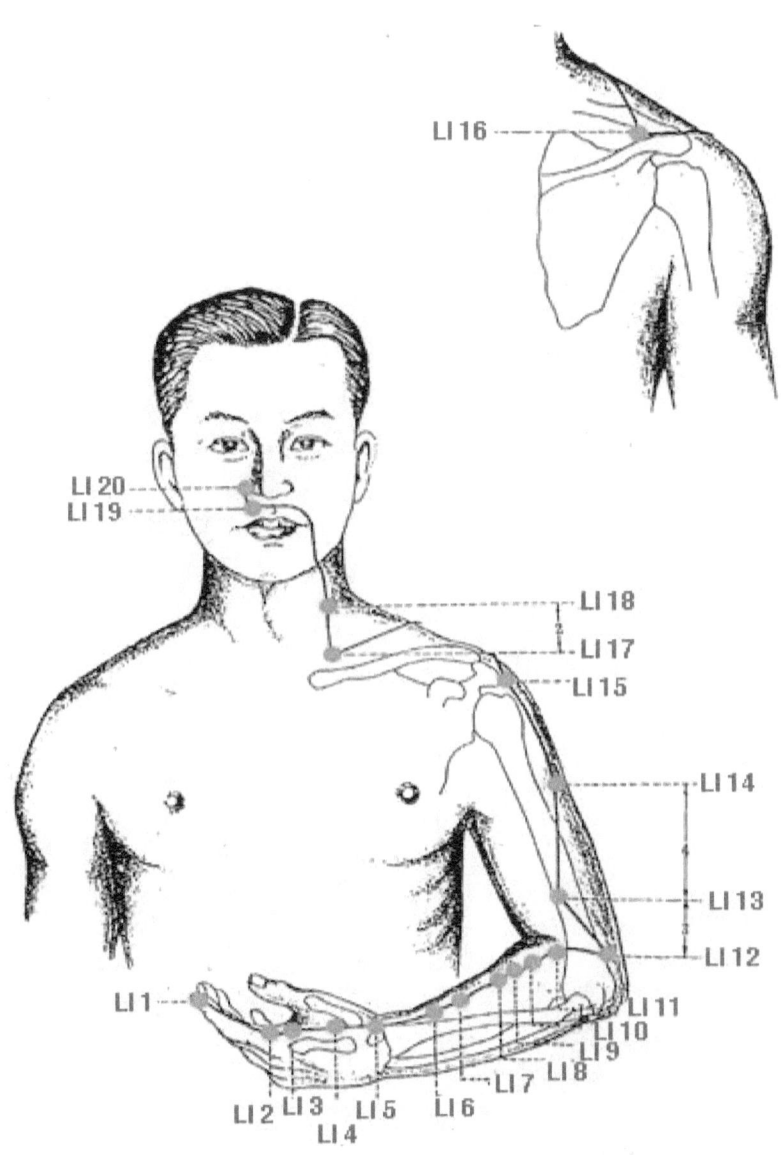

⊛ **IG: Intestino grueso**

Nombre:

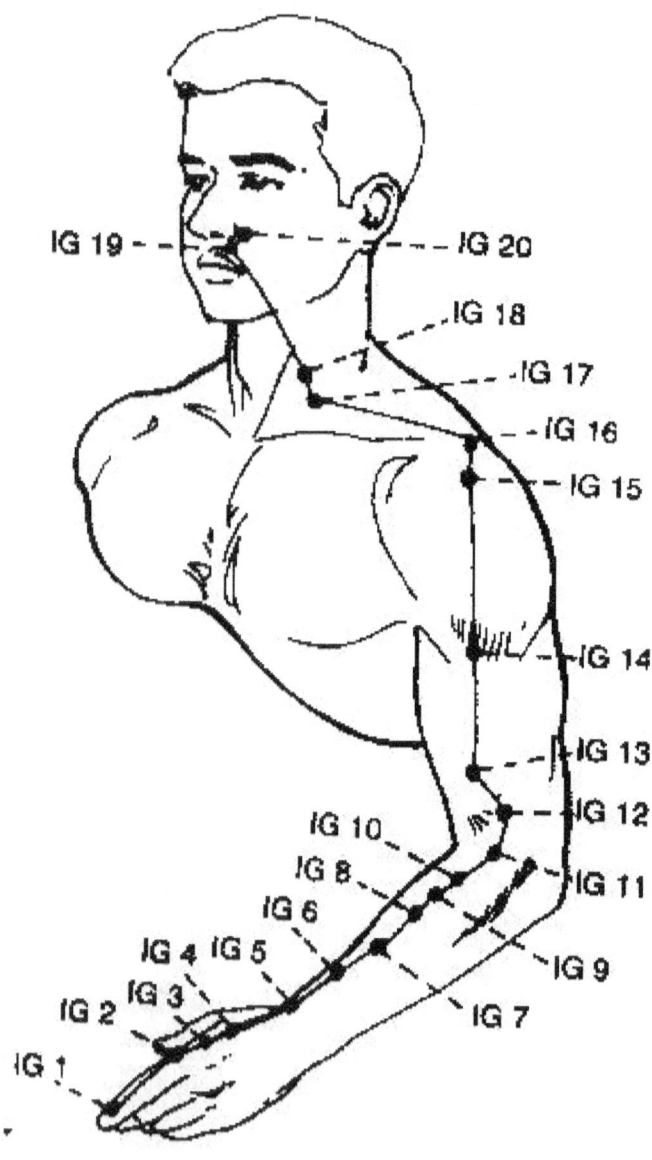

⚜ TH: TRIPLE HEATER

Name:

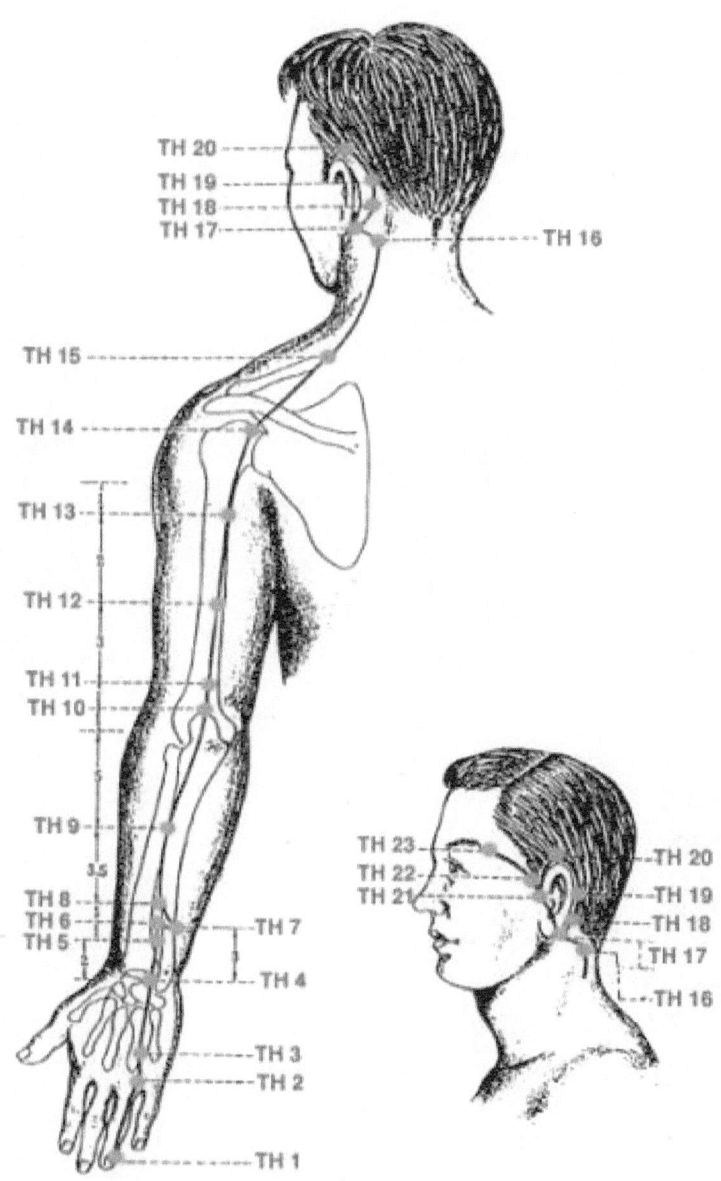

125

🐝 TR: Triple recalentador

Nombre:

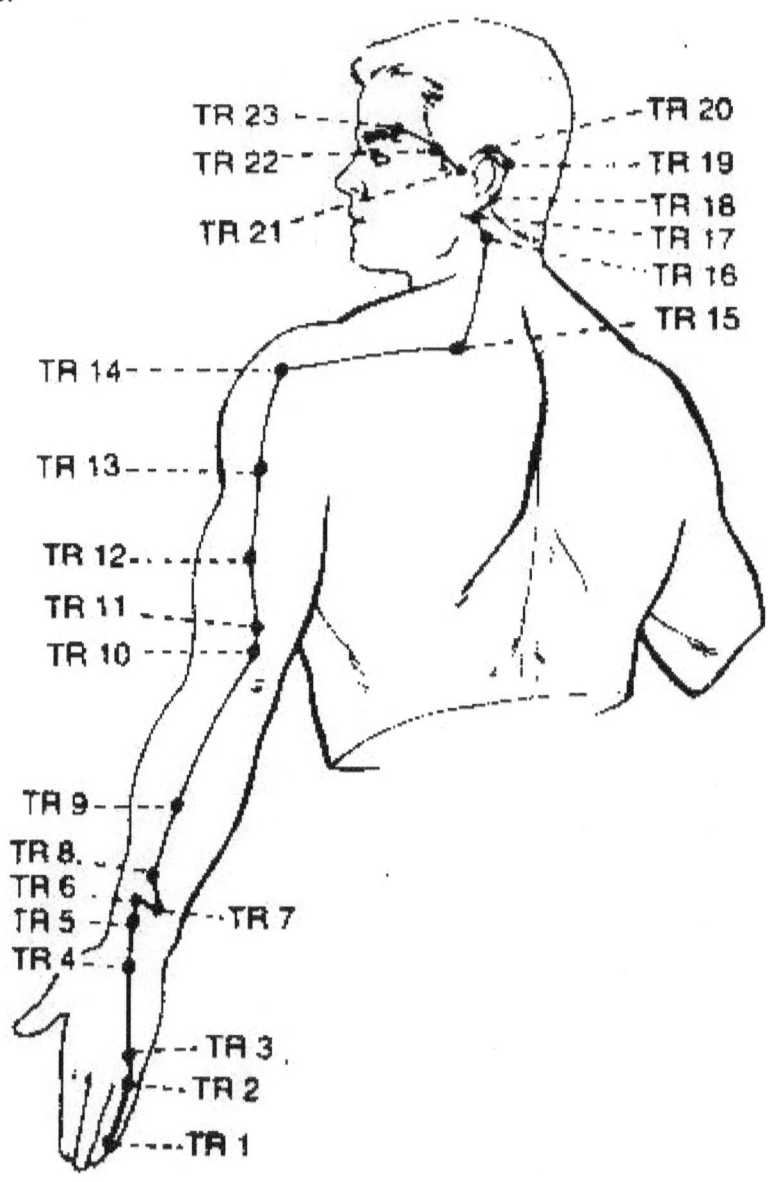

⚕ ST: STOMACH

Name:

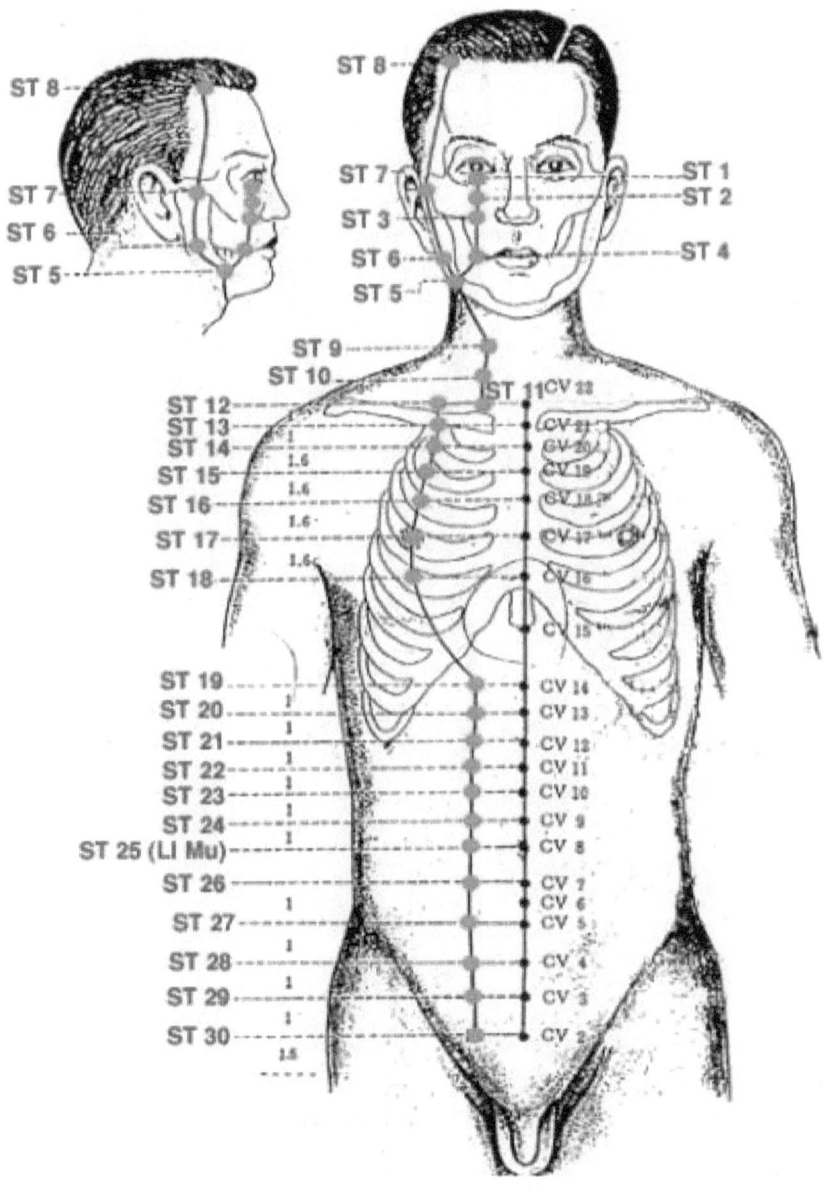

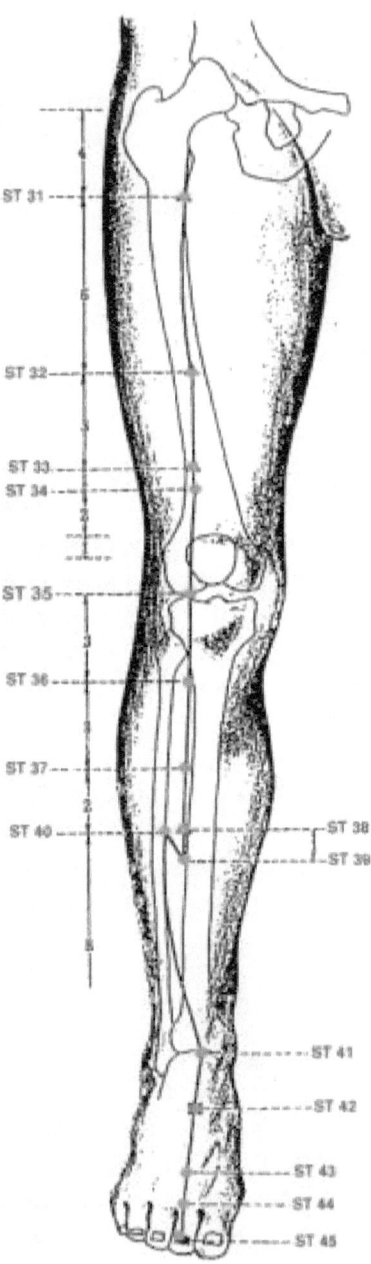

⊛ **E: Estómago**

Nombre:

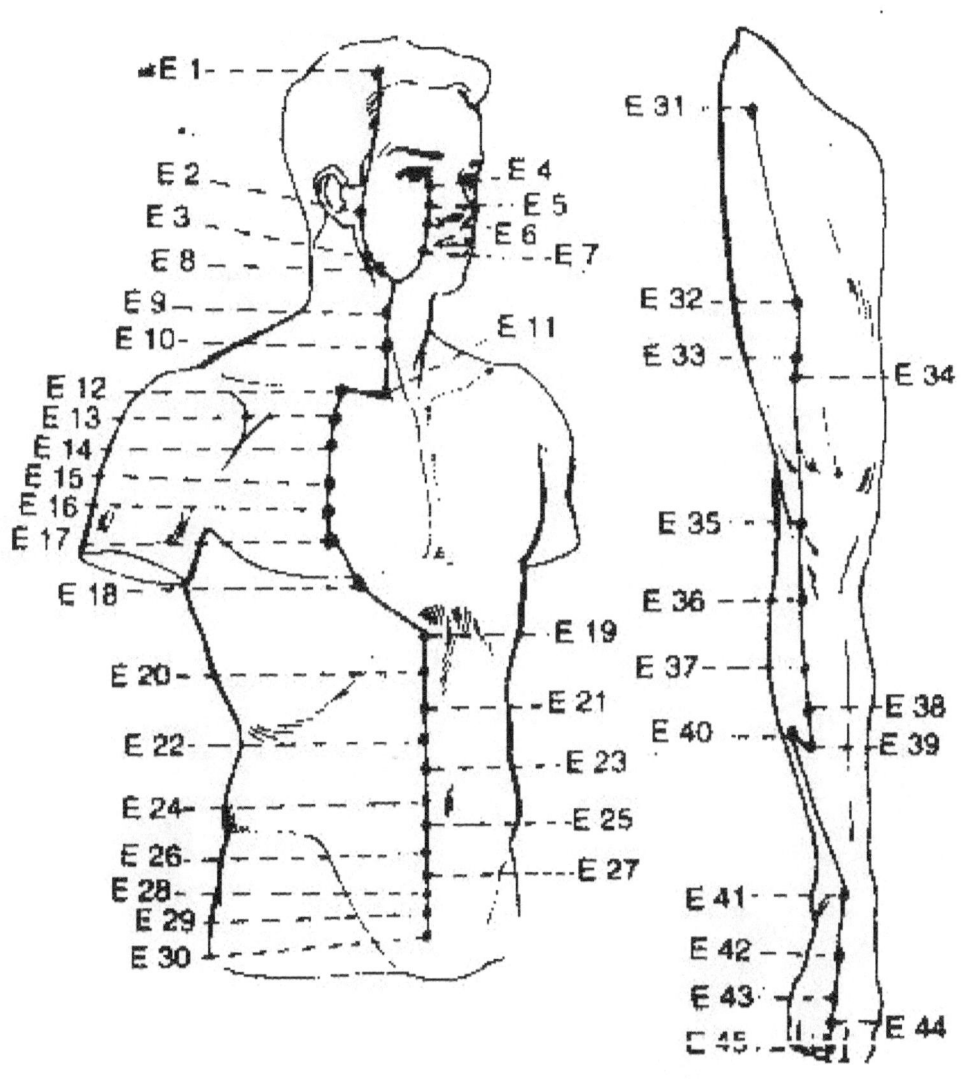

⊛ UB: URINARY BLADDER

Name:

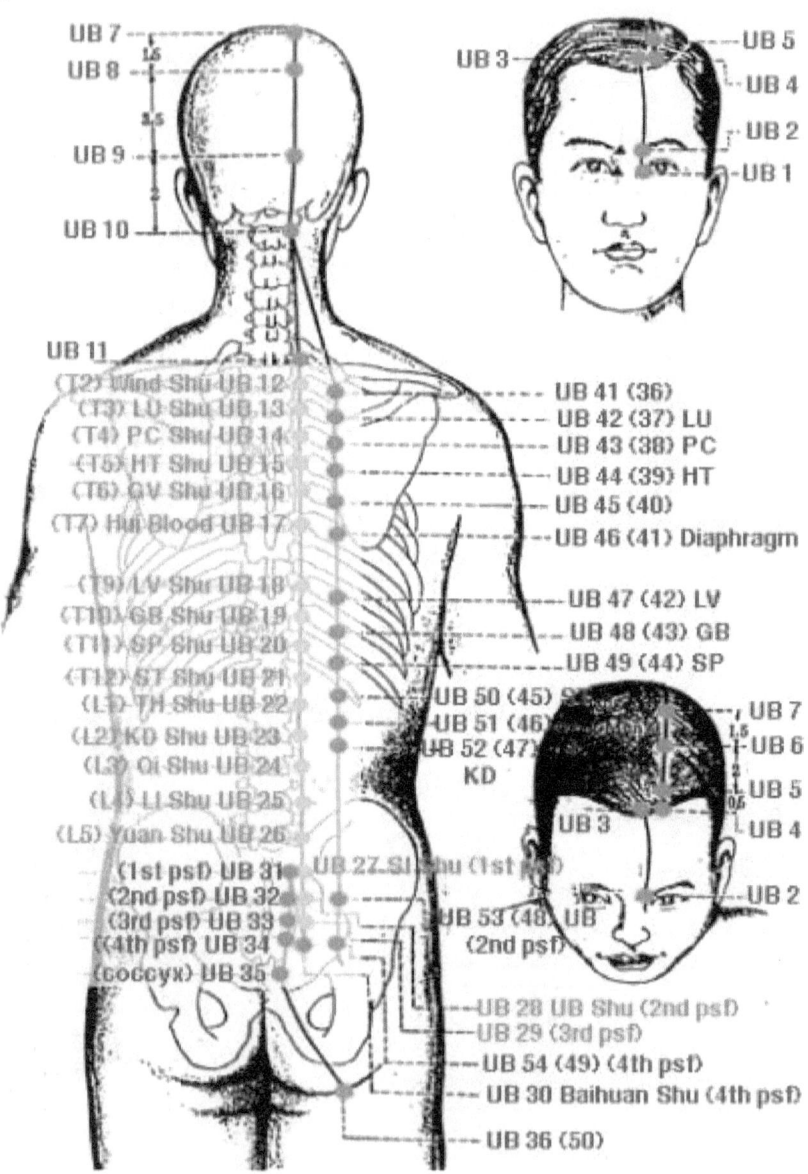

UB 7
UB 8
1.5
3.5
UB 9
UB 10

UB 3
UB 5
UB 4
UB 2
UB 1

UB 11
(T2) Wind Shu UB 12
(T3) LU Shu UB 13
(T4) PC Shu UB 14
(T5) HT Shu UB 15
(T6) GV Shu UB 16
(T7) Hui Blood UB 17

UB 41 (36)
UB 42 (37) LU
UB 43 (38) PC
UB 44 (39) HT
UB 45 (40)
UB 46 (41) Diaphragm

(T9) LV Shu UB 18
(T10) GB Shu UB 19
(T11) SP Shu UB 20
(T12) ST Shu UB 21
(L1) TH Shu UB 22
(L2) KD Shu UB 23
(L3) Qi Shu UB 24
(L4) LI Shu UB 25
(L5) Yuan Shu UB 26

UB 47 (42) LV
UB 48 (43) GB
UB 49 (44) SP
UB 50 (45)
UB 51 (46)
UB 52 (47) KD

UB 7
UB 6
UB 5
UB 4
1.5
0.5

UB 3
UB 2

(1st psf) UB 31
(2nd psf) UB 32
(3rd psf) UB 33
(4th psf) UB 34
(coccyx) UB 35

UB 27 SI Shu (1st psf)
UB 53 (48) UB (2nd psf)

UB 28 UB Shu (2nd psf)
UB 29 (3rd psf)
UB 54 (49) (4th psf)
UB 30 Baihuan Shu (4th psf)
UB 36 (50)

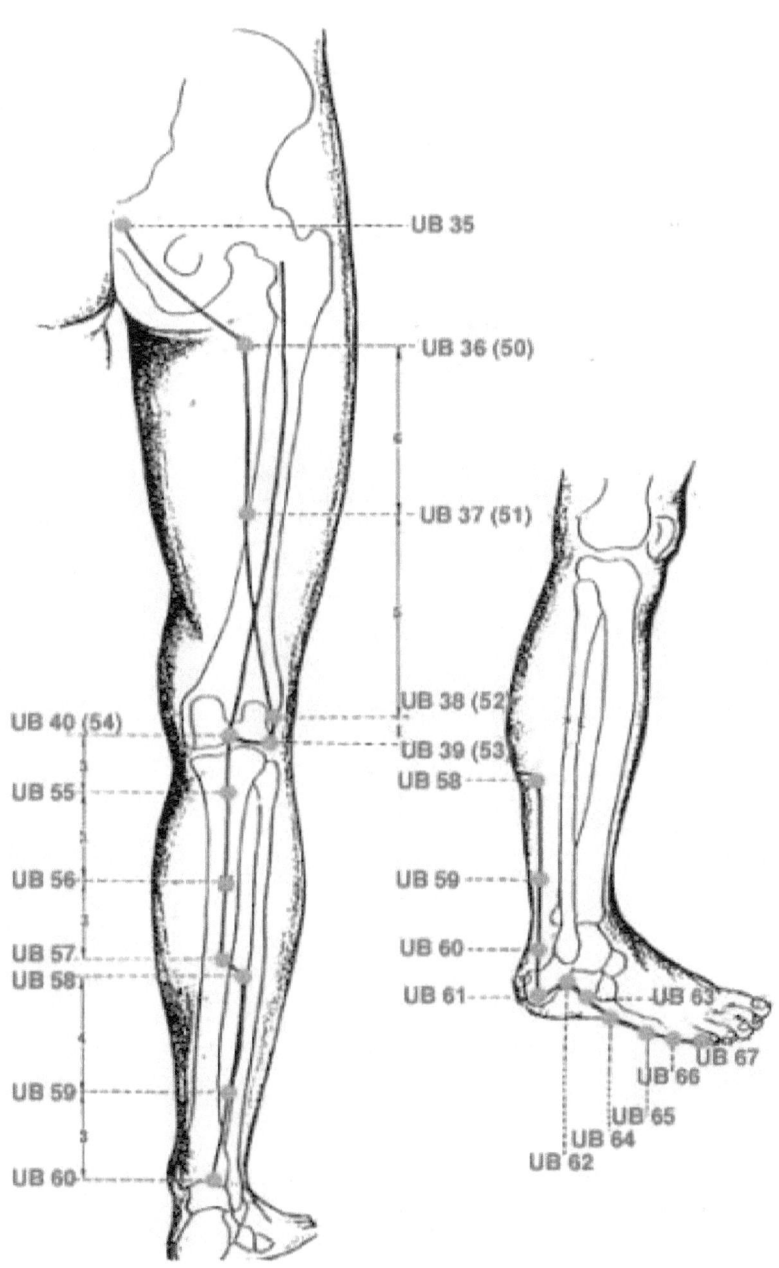

🐝 V: Vejiga

Nombre:

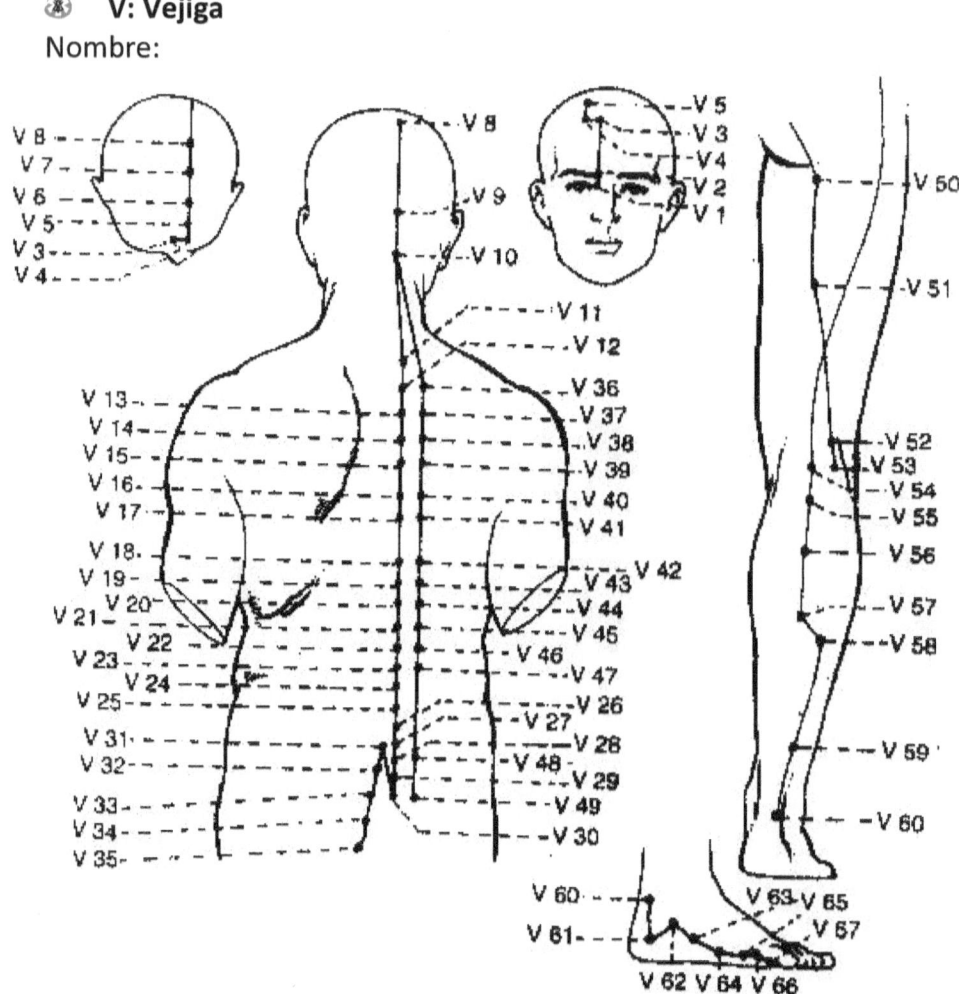

⚘ GB: GALL BLADDER

Name

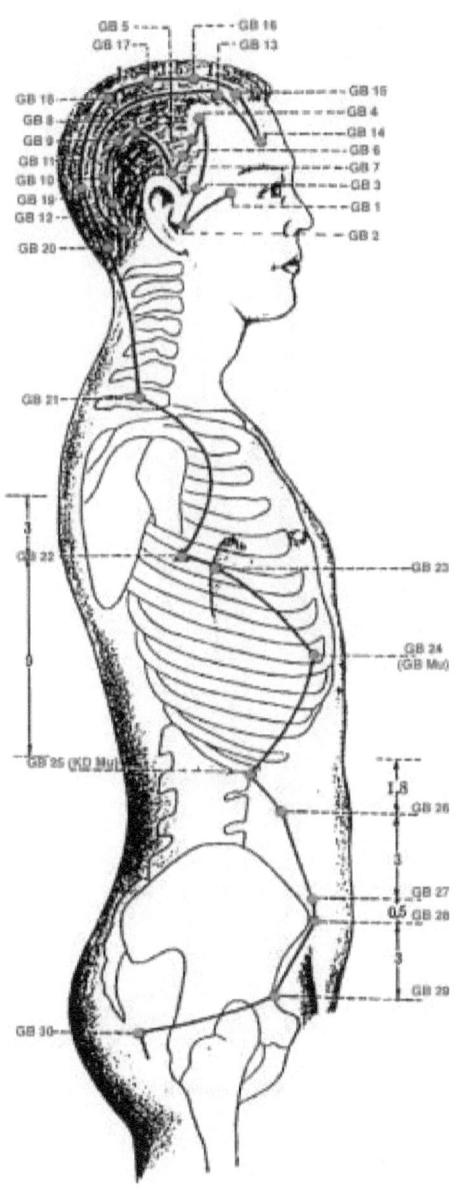

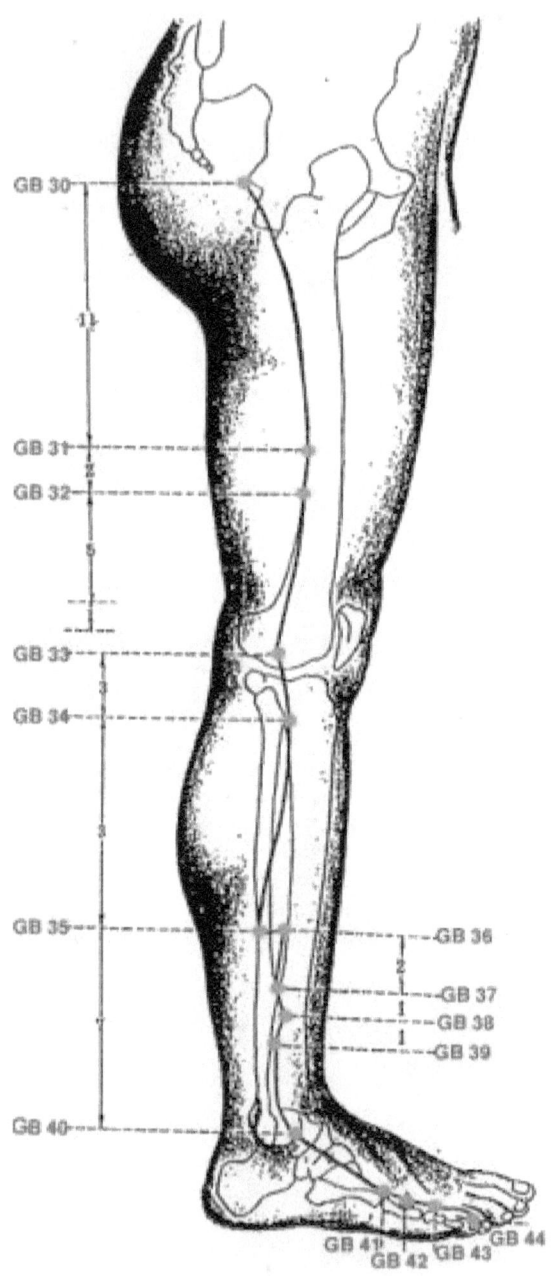

❀ VB: Vesícula biliar

Nombre:

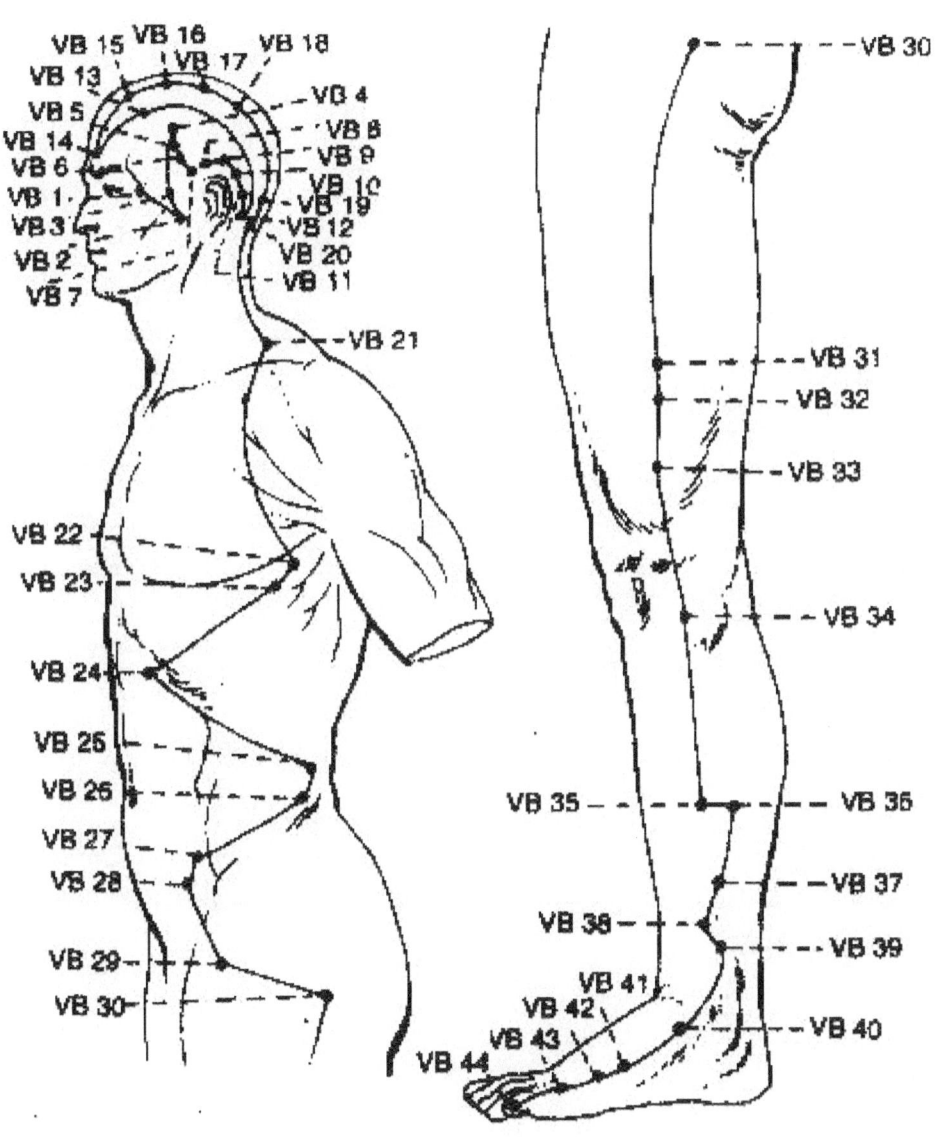

NOTES

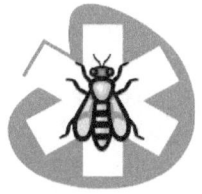

12. NATIONAL APITHERAPY SOCIETIES

ARGENTINA: Asociación Argentina de Apiterapia (Argentinian Apitherapy Association), Avenida Agustín Álvarez 1368, Zona Rural Paraje El Chaja, Partido 9 de Julio, Provincia de Buenos Aires, Argentina. ✉ info@aadapiterapia.com.ar. 🖥 www.aadapiterapia.com.ar.

AUSTRALIA: Australian Apitherapy Association, 8 Kennedy Road, Bli Bli, Queensland 4560, Australia. ☎ 61(75) 450-0624. ✉ info@apitherapy.org.au. 🖥 www.apitherapy.org.au.

AUSTRALIA: Australian Apitherapy Society, P.O. Box H221, Australia Square, Sydney NSW 1215, Australia. ☎ 61(2)8904-9162. ✉ gzachary@bigpond.net.au.

AUSTRIA: Österreichische Gesellschaft für Apitherapie (Austrian Apitherapy Society). 🖥 www.apitherapie.at.

BRAZIL: Sociedade Brasileira de Apiterapia (Brazilian Apitherapy Society). 🖥 www.sbaapiterapia.com.br.

BRAZIL: Associação Paulista de Apicultores e Criadores de Abelhas Melíficas Européias (APACAME), Parque da Água Branca, Casa do Fazendeiro, Térreo, Ave. Francisco Matarazzo 455, 05001-300 São Paulo SP, Brasil. ☎ 55(11)3864-9284. ✉ apacame@apacame.org.br. 🖥 www.apacame.org.br.

BULGARIA: Bulgarian Apitherapy Union, Kosta Lultchev 5, Bloc 128, 1113 Sofia, Bulgaria. ☎ 35(92)705-867. ✉ bankova@orgchm.bas.bg.

CANADA: Canadian Apitherapy Association / Association Canadienne d'Apitherapie. 🖥 www.canadian-apitherapy-association.ca.

CHILE: Asociación Chilena de Apiterapeutas (Chilean Association of Apitherapists), 1985 Errazuriz 30, Buin, Santiago, Chile. ✆ 56(652)259-0873. ✉ jaraneda@achia.cl. ⌨ www.achia.cl.

CHINA: Apitherapy Department of the Chinese Beekeeping Association, Fuzhou, Fujian Province, China. ✉ harmony_mj@126.com.

CHINA: International Apitherapy Healthcare and Bee Acupuncture Association, Wen-hao Garden # 79, Nanking Lukou, Jiangsu 211113, China. ✆ 86(25)245-0865. ✉ iahbafz@jlonline.com.

COLOMBIA: Sociedad Colombiana de Apiterapia (Colombian Apitherapy Society). ⌨ www.apiterapiacolombia.com.co.

CZECH REPUBLIC: Česká Apiterapeutická Společnost (Czech Apitherapy Society). ✉ info@capis.cz. ⌨ www.capis.cz.

ECUADOR: Sociedad Ecuatoriana de Apiterapia (Ecuatorian Apitherapy Association), Diego de Vacas N77-30 y Clemente Yerovi, Quito, Ecuador. ✆ 59(32)510-1251. ⌨ http://apiterapia.com.ec.

EGYPT: Bee Venom Therapy Research Center. ⌨www.beevenomcenter .com.

EGYPT: Egyptian Society of Apitherapy and Egyptian Environmental Society for Uses and Production of Bee Products, National Research Center, Dokki, Giza, Egypt. ✆ 20(2)774-9222. ✉ ahmedhegazi128 @gmail.com. ⌨ www.ahmedhegazi.com.

FRANCE: Association Francophone d'Apithérapie. ⌨ www.apitherapie-francophone.com.

FRANCE: Association Francophone d'Apithérapie et Phytothérapie. ⌨ www.api-phytotherapie.fr.

GERMANY: Deutscher Apitherapie Bund (German Apitherapy Society), Weidenbachring 14, 82362 Weilheim-Marnbach, Germany. ✆ 49 (881) 9245-1395. ⌨ www.apitherapie.de.

GREECE: Greek Scientific Apitherapy Center, Chryson 7, Acharnai, 13671 Attica,Greece. ✆ 30(210)246-5021. ✉ joanmag@vodafone.net.gr.

HUNGARY: Magyar Apiterápiás Társaság (Hungarian Apitherapy Soci- ety), Széna utca 7, Nagykovácsi 2094 Budapest, Hungary. ✆ 36(30)948-6635. ▭ www.apiterapia.hu.

INDONESIA: Yayasan Terapi Lebah Indonesia (Indonesia Apitherapy Foundation), Graha Sucofindo, Gedung D, Lantai Dasar, Jl. Raya Ps. Minggu Kav. 34, Jakarta, Indonesia. ✆ 62(21)7918-8323. ✉ info@api -therapy-indonesia.com. ▭ www.apitherapy-indonesia.com.

INTERNATIONAL FEDERATION OF APITHERAPY:
▭ www.api-terra.org.

ISRAEL: Israeli Apitherapy Centre. ✆972(50)787-5543. ▭ www.apitherapy.co.il.

ITALY: Associazione Italiana di Apiterapia (Italian Apitherapy Association). ✉ info@apiterapiaitalia.com, segreteria@apiterapiaitalia.com. ▭ www.apiterapiaitalia.com, https://apiterapiablog.wordpress.com.

JAPAN: Japan Apitherapy Association, Muyukimachi 6-3-26, Sizunai-machi, Sizunai-gun, Hokkaido, Japan. ✆ 81(14)642-2618. ▭ www.- apithera-jp.com.

JAPAN: Propolis Researchers Association, Honeybee Science Research Center, Tamagawa University, Machida-shi, Tokyo 194-8610, Japan. ✆ 81(42)739-8685. ▭ www.tamagawa.ac.jp/HSRC/index.html.

KOREA: Korean Apitherapy and Healthcare Association, Sinsang- ri 1059 – 2 (c/o Koryo Apiary), Jinryang-ub, Gyeongsan-si, Gyeongsangbuk-do 712 – 837, Korea. ▭ www.apitherapy.co.kr

LITHUANIA: Lithuanian Apitherapy Association, Zariju Str. 2B, LT-02053 Vilnius, Lithuania.✆371(7)225-231. ✉ sonatai@centras.lt; apiterapija.lt@gmail.com; pov.rimkus@gmail.com. ▭ www.apiterapija.lt.

MALAYSIA: Malaysian Association of Apitherapy, 28-3, Persiaran 65C, Off Jalan Pahang Barat, 53000 Kuala Lumpur, West Malaysia. ✆ 012-455-7897. ✉ penangapis@myjaring.net. 🖥 www.beeacupuncture.org.

MALAYSIA: Malaysian Apitherapy Society, c/o Dept. of Pharmacology, School of Medical Sciences, Health Campus, Universiti Sains Malaysia, 15150 Kubang Kerian, Kelantan, Malaysia.

MEXICO: Sociedad Mexicana de Apiterapia (Mexican Apitherapy Society). 🖥 www.apiterapiamexicana.mx.

PERU: Asociación Peruana de Apiterapia (Peruvian Apitherapy Association), Centro de Apiterapia, Centro Comercial la Rotonda II Etapa, Oficina 1062, La Molina, Lima, Perú. ✆ 51(14)349-7564. ✉ informes@inkasbees.com. 🖥 www.inkasbees.com.

PORTUGAL: Associação Portuguesa de Apiterapia (Portuguese Apitherapy Association), Bairro do Alvito 9, 1300-052 Lisbon, Portugal. ✆ 35(193)802-5330. 🖥 www.apiterapia.pt.

ROMANIA: Societatea Romana de Apiterapie (Romanian Apitherapy Society), Strada Nucilor Nr. 3, oras Magurele, jud. Ilfov, 077125 Romania. ✉ secretariat@apiterapie.ro. 🖥 www.apiterapie.ro.

SERBIA: Srpsko Apiterapeutsko Društvo (Serbian Apitherapy Society), Daniciceva St. No. 7, 18000 Nis, Serbia. ✆ 38(11) 856-2574. ✉ vericamilojkovic@yahoo.com.

SLOVENIA: Slovenian Apitherapy Department of the Slovenian Beekeepers' Association (Čebelarska Zveza Slovenije), Brdo 8, 1225 Ludovica, Slovenia. ✆ 38(61) 7296-100. ✉ info@czs.si. 🖥 www.czs.si. *Slovenski Čevelar.*

SPAIN: Asociación Española e Internacional de Apiterapia (Spanish and International Apitherapy Association). ✆ 34(661)81-0310.

SPAIN: Sociedad Española de Apiterapeutas (Spanish Society of Apitherapists). ✆ 34(695)38-6714.

SWITZERLAND: Schweizerischer Apitherapie Verein / Association Suisse d'Apithérapie (Swiss Apitherapy Society). 🏦 infof@apitherapie.ch.   ⬚ www.apitherapie.ch (German language), www.apitherapie-fr.ch (French language).

TAIWAN: Taiwan Apitherapy Association, 108-8, Ain-Si Road, Chang-Hua City, 500 Taiwan. 📞 88(64)738-1524. 🏦 harrisonip@netscape.net.

TURKEY: Apiterapi Dernegi-Balnak (Turkish Apitherapy Society), Merkez Mahallesi Dereboyu Caddesi No. 56, Halkali – Küçükçekmece TR-34303 Istanbul, Turkey. 📞 90 (212) 473-1515. 🏦 info@apiterapidernegi.org.

UKRAINE: Ukrainian Association of Apitherapists. ⬚ apispilka.in.ua

UNITED KINGDOM: United Kingdom Apitherapy Society, 37 Cecil Road, Cheshunt, Herts EN8 8TN, United Kingdom. 📞 44 (199) 262-2645. 🏦 peter.pebadale@virgin.net.   ⬚   http://freespace-virgin.net/peter.pebadale/pages/UK_Api_Society.htm#UK.

UNITED STATES: American Apitherapy Society, 500 Arthur Street, Centerport, NY 11721, USA. 📞 1(631)470-9446. 🏦 aasoffice@ apitherapy.org. ⬚ www.apitherapy.org. *Journal of the American Apitherapy Society.*

VENEZUELA: Asociación Venezolana de Apiterapia (Venezuelan Apitherapy Association). 📞 58(274)808-4106. ⬚ www.ava.com.ve (http: //archive.is/vU65L).

 For additional information on Apitherapy societies: www.apitherapy.com/api-countries-addresses and other internet sites. Information on Apitherapy societies frequently changes and it is a good opportunity to use the Notes/Notas available in prior and next pages.

Bees for Life
World Apitherapy Network

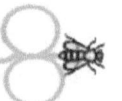

Beekeepers and Apitherapists Without Borders
Apicultores e Apiterapeutas Sem Fronteiras
Imkern und Apitherapeuten Ohne Grenzen
Apiculteurs et Apithérapeutes Sans Frontières
Apicultores y Apiterapeutas Sin Fronteras

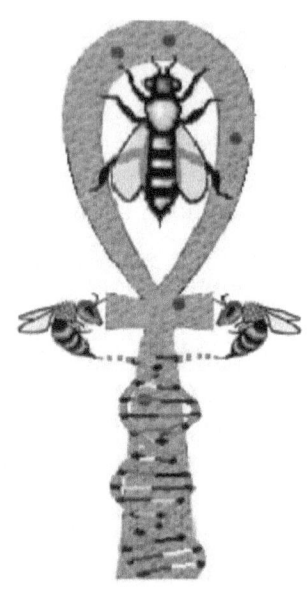

A nonprofit charitable, scientific and educational organization, **Bees for Life—World Apitherapy** Inc. was created in 2005 under Section 501(c)(3) of 1986 Code of Internal Revenue Service, to assist "victims of famine, epidemics, disasters, wars, and other events affecting public health and needy populations" (Articles of Incorporation, § VII.5, document N05000012210 of Florida State Department, EIN 20-3703789 of IRS).

It was supported by thousands of volunteers around the world, who intervened with their skills in Apitherapy and beekeeping for assisting victims of earthquakes, hurricanes, epidemics, war scenarios, and for outreach and education in all countries. A hundred percent of its operations in Miami and elsewhere were funded by some donations and the royalties from Apitherapy books, but in 2016 the organization couldn't cope longer with the annual government fees and the minimal operational expenses and, once funds were totally exhausted, it made the decision to continue its activities as a group in Facebook:

www.Facebook.com/groups/BeesForLifeWorldApitherapy

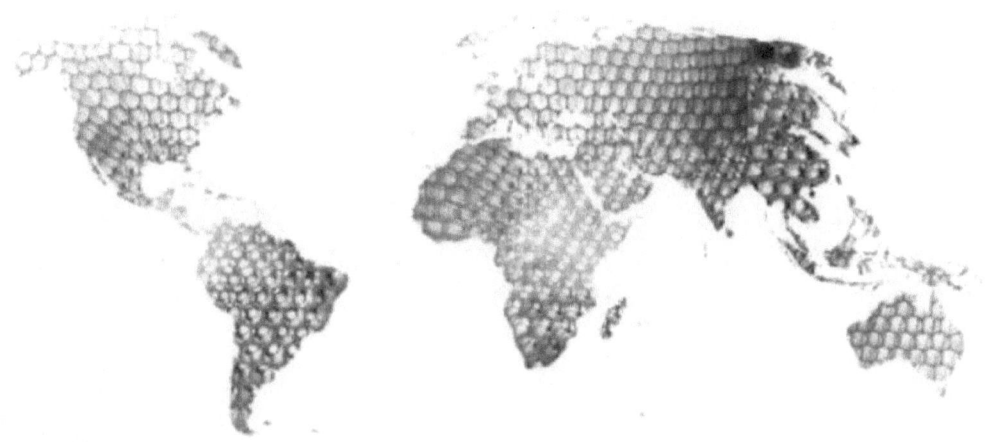

NOTES

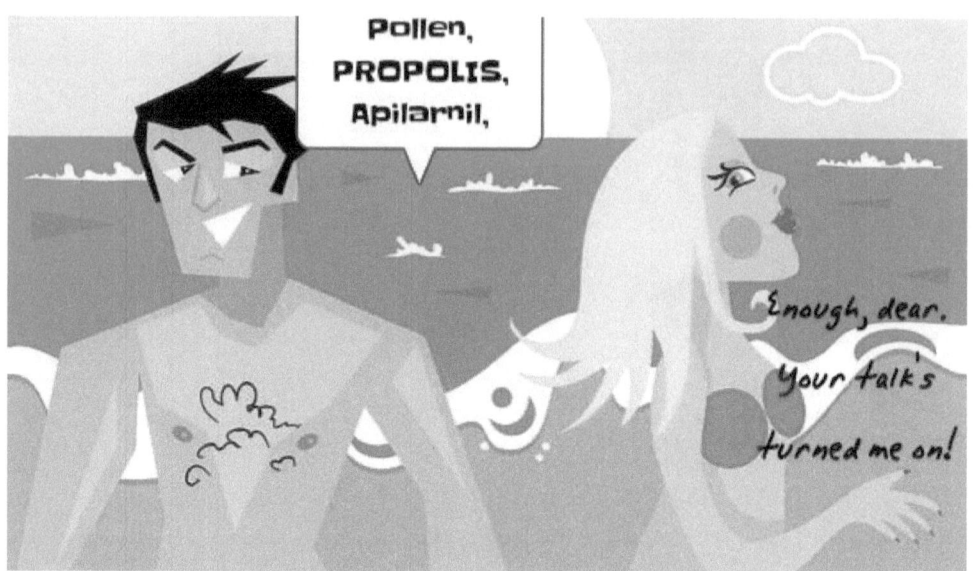

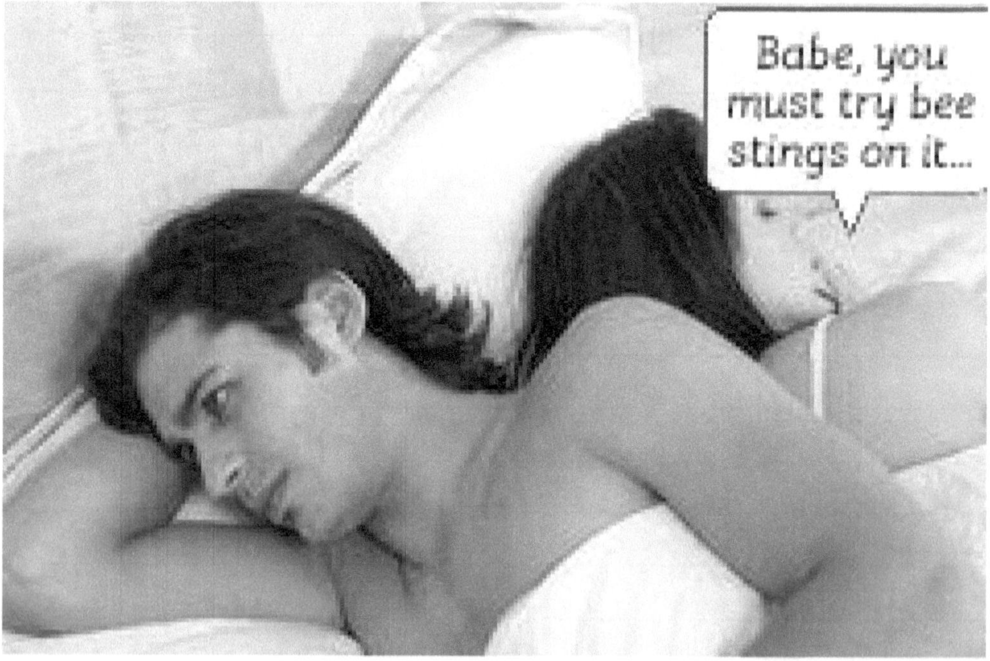

World Apitherapy Day

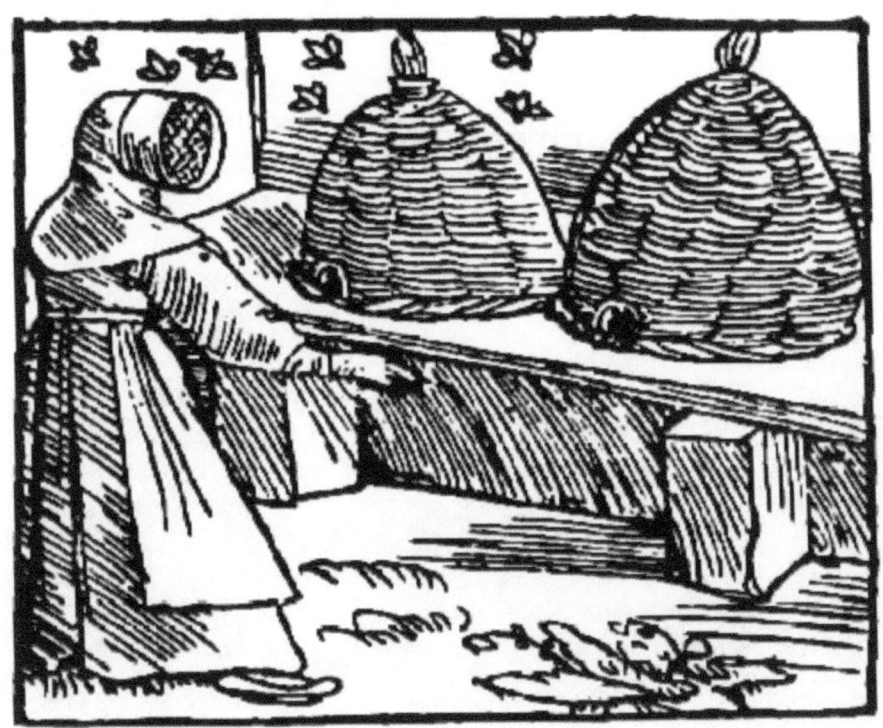

世界蜂針研究天

Día Mundial de la Apiterapia

اليوم العالمي للعلاج بمنتجات النحل

Мировой день апитерапии

Journée mondiale de l'apithérapie

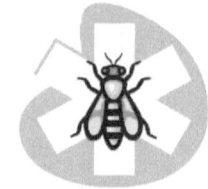

13. WORLD APITHERAPY DAY

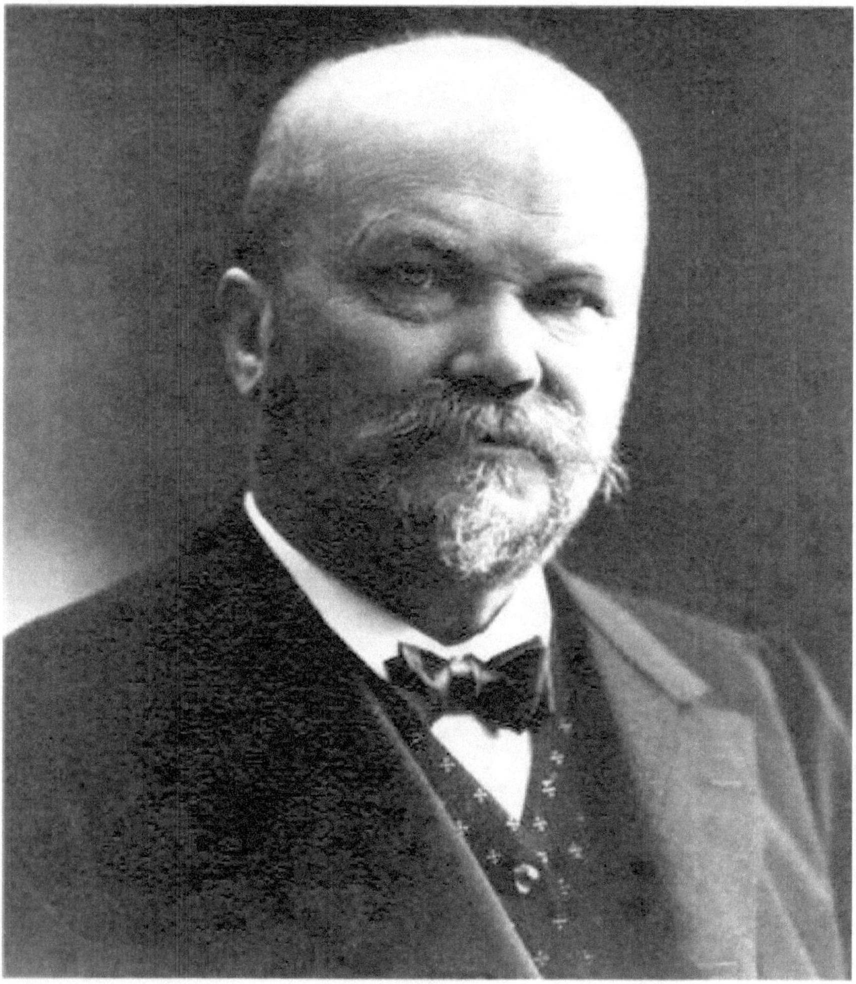

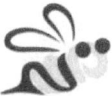

Filip Terč (1844 - 1917) and the birth of Apitherapy

The first time someone used the term "Apitherapy" it was to explain the medical use of bee stings or Apitoxitherapy.

This historical mention doesn't imply that other apitherapeutic products have not a very ancient background. On the contrary, medicinal uses of hive products are mentioned in Ebers papyrus (1700 BCE), *Torah* (*Gen.*37.25 & 43.11), *The Prophets* and other Biblical books (*Jer.* 8.22, 46.11, 51.8. *Prov.* 24.13, & *1Sam.* 14.25-29), in the works by Aristotle, Pliny, Dioscorides, Galen, Hippocrates, Varro, Avicenna and other ancient scholars which trace all background on Apitherapy, and in *Vedas* and *Quran*, the therapy field of bee products. It was in the Bible that I found some first references to propolis (צרי *tzori*). In the case of apitoxin, diverse uses were known in different centuries and there are references, for example, to the healing of chronic gout suffered by Charlemagne (748 – 814) and the relief of join pain suffered by Ivan IV the Terrible (1530 – 1584) thanks to increasing number of bee stings. However, I want to shortly emphasize the applications of apitoxin from a difficult and transforming period of the history of Medicine: the 19th Century.

In that century, historians underlined the example of a physician, Ignác Fülöp Semmelweis, pioneer of antisepsis. I remember that one of my first childhood readings was a Semmelweis biography, and never forgot that hero of science who unutterably suffered while trying to convince his colleagues that it was possible to save thousands of women's lives who had died from puerperal fever. When he started working in 1847 at the obstetrical department of University of Vienna, maternal mortality was 26 %. Semmelweis suggested once and again that the cause for that high mortality was the puerperal sepsis originated from doctors not washing their hands after manipulating corpses. Once and again, academic authorities rejected his opinion regardless of his victories in reducing maternal mortality to a low 0.5 % at Vienna General Hospital in 1860.

Semmelweis couldn't overcome the opposition to his solid statements. In 1865, at 47 years old and after several years suffering from an early-type or presenile dementia, his own family and friends placed him at the Niederösterreichische

Landesirrenaustalt, a private nursing home in Vienna, where he suffered from violence outbursts and two weeks later died from the beatings by psychiatric ward's staff. A few years afterwards, physician Joseph Lister advocated for surgical antisepsis methods, praising Semmelweis's contributions, and for that reason Lister is today's father of antiseptic surgery.

There are many similarities between the life of Filip Terč, "Father of Modern Apitherapy", and Semmelweis's biography. Terč was a teenager when Semmelweis discovered the prophylaxis method and was losing his battle for the truth. As some historical coincidences –already pointed out by physician Bodog Beck-, both scientists had the same first name in German (Philipp), and both were physicians who had to face a similar academic dogmatism in nineteenth-century Vienna.

Terč was born on March 30, 1844 in Prapořiště (former Braunpusch), a tiny village in Czech region of western Bohemia. At that time Bohemia was a part of Austrian Empire and in 1867 to 1918 a part of the Austro-Hungarian Empire. Terč was the son of Johann Tertsch and Barbara Stepan, and his original family name was Tertsch, according to Plzeň State Archives (tome 12, folio 8).

Terč suffered from rheumatism and had intense joint pain, and nothing he could try would bring him relief, despite his role as a prestigious general practitioner in Maribor (Marburg an der Drau), southeastern extreme of the Duchy of Lower Styria, also a part of the Austro-Hungarian Empire. One day in 1868 a group of bees suddenly stung him and, to his surprise, from then on, his pain began to disappear and his limbs recovered more mobility. This personal experience impressed him which led him to consider that the clinical studies in France in 1859 by a physician Desjardins, and in Russia in 1864 by a physician M.I. Lukomsky on the therapeutic effects of bee stings should have been taken seriously and ought to be submitted to scientific research.

Only until eleven years later did he seriously take interest in researching the cause of his amazing cure. A female patient had been treated by different doctors and even by Terč for a severe cranial neuralgia and deafness, and even the most advanced medical procedures had been fruitless. Then the lady asked Terč for any new procedures, as she felt disappointed for her lack of recovery. Terč remembered his own experiences and all his readings on the effect of bee venom. He then proceeded apply daily bee stings, up to 90 bee stings a day, with no improvement in her condition, however he did notice that stings didn't also bring any negative effect. One day he applied 15 bee stings on her neck and shoulders and, surprise, the woman was totally cured from neuralgia and deafness, but for the first time since the start of treatment her face was swollen from the stings.

Terč continued his observations and experiments for the following 10 years and, in 1889, he presented to the University of Vienna his outstanding conclusions about thousands of patients successfully treated. Unfortunately, he faced a hostile and intransigent audience, to the point that Terč decided to leave Vienna out of fear for being interned in a psychiatric ward. The University of Vienna used to publish all conferences given by guest scientists, but Terč's conference was never published. Contempt suffered in the past and later by Franz Anton Mesmer, Louis Pasteur, Philipp Semmelweis, Edward Jenner, Carlos J. Finlay, Nikola Tesla, and many others, was being repeated now with Terč, who took the decision of returning to Maribor in order to inconspicuously continue his treatments with apitoxin.

As a testimonial on his research work, he left several publications as well as a book published in 1910. In his *Report on the peculiar connection between bee stings and rheumatism* (1888), Terč describes his treatment of 660 patients suffering from rheumatic arthritis and applied to them a total of 39,000 bee stings: 82 % had a perfect cure (544 patients), 15 % had recovery (99 patients) and only 3 % had no relief (17 patients).

In 1914, Alfred Keiter, MD, published in Vienna and Leipzig a book describing Terč's research works: *Rheumatismus and Bienen- stichbehandlung; Der heutige Stand derselben mit einem Beitrage von Dr. Philipp Terč*. One of Terč's sons, Rudolf Tertsch, ophtalmologist in Vienna, published a book in 1912 describing his father's research, *Das Bienengift im Dienste der Medizin*, and Terč's grandson, Rudolf Tertsch, a doctor in Meerbusch and deceased in 1982, continued the family tradition of applying bee stings to his patients.

In 2006, after an initiative from nonprofit organization Bees for Life – World Apitherapy Network Inc., for the first time March 30 was celebrated in Prapořiště as the "World Apitherapy Day", to honor pioneer scientific research by Filip Terč, "Father of Modern Apitherapy", and his professional integrity.

Honors have been paid to Terč in 2015 in Maribor, Slovenia, where he has his grave, and on October 28, 2017 the centenary of his decease was commemorated in his birth town in the Czech Republic.

In 1935, in his unequaled book *Bee venom therapy*, Bodog F. Beck, MD (1871 - 1942), for the first time used the term Apitherapy to describe bee venom therapy. Beck was born in Hungary and brought to the United States the best from European knowledge on Apitherapy and inspired many other people to continue his work, specially Charles Mraz (1905 - 1999), who promoted the creation of the American Apitherapy Society (www.apitherapy.org) and motivated, altogether with many colleagues from America, Europe, and other latitudes, the present development of Apitherapy as a branch of Complementary and Alternative Medicine.

Each day the use of bee venom becomes more and more widely employed in the treatment of many disorders, and dozens of branded apitoxin products are marketed by beekeepers and the pharmaceutical industry. But furthermore, 14 other beehive products including honey, propolis, bee pollen, mead, bee bread, honeydew honey, drone larvae, géopropolis, royal jelly, beeswax, whole bees, honeycomb capping, hive air, and stingless bee honey, are presently used and researched for therapeutic use.

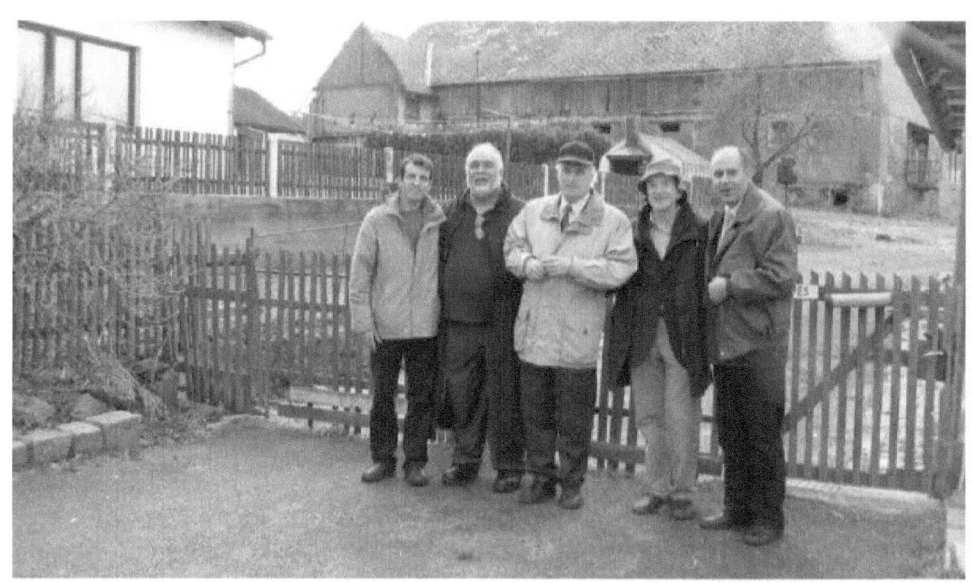

The first celebration of World Apitherapy Day on March 30, 2006, in Prapořiště. A barn in the background and three contiguous old houses belonged to Filip Terč's family and here he was born. In the picture, the founders of Bees for Life (left to right) Antonio Couto (Portugal), Moisés Asís (USA), Pedro Pérez (Spain), and Ştefan Stângaciu (Romania), with Jan Löffelman (at the center), Kdyně District Mayor.

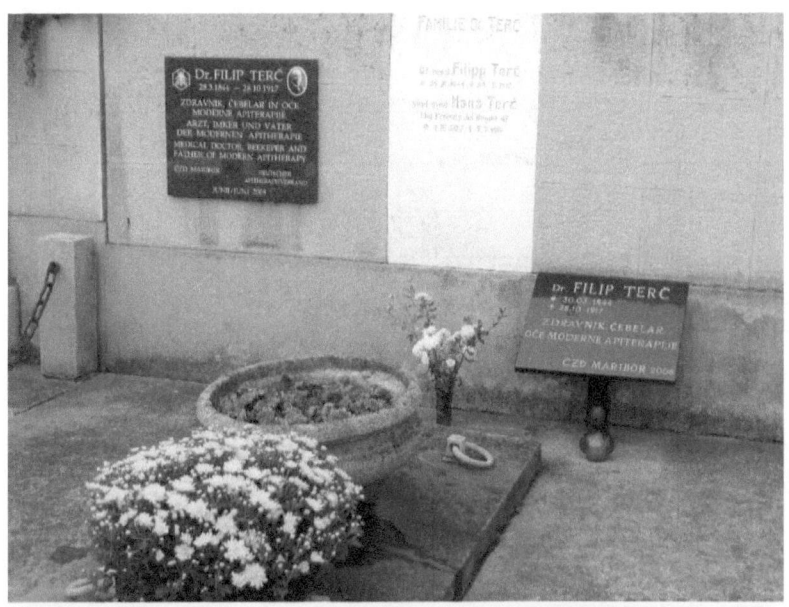

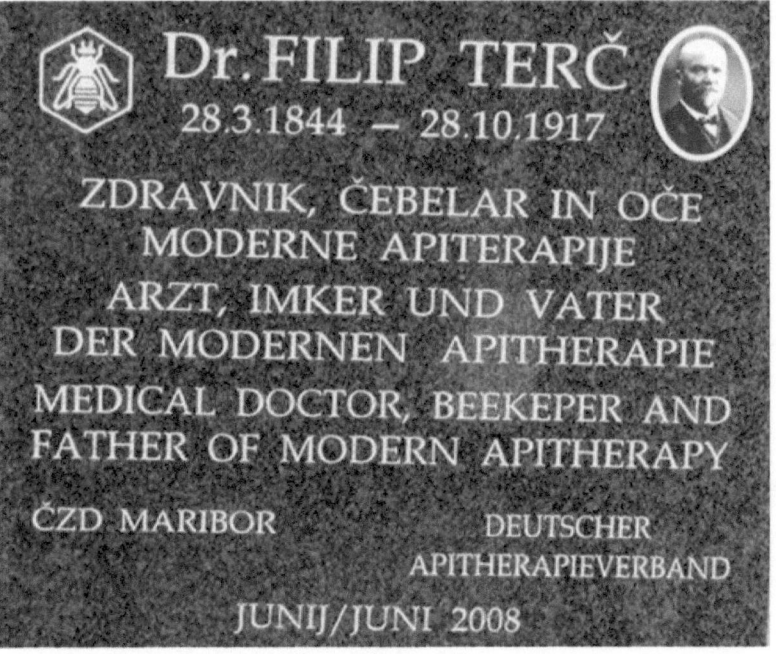

Gravesite of Filip Terč in Pokopališče Pobrežje (Maribor cemetery), in Slovenia.

NOTES

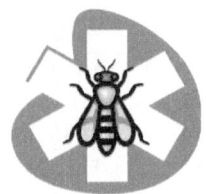

14. WORLD EMERGENCY NUMBERS

Just in case, as Apitherapy becomes widely used worldwide, although rare, an anaphylactic reaction or accident could happen if proper precautions are not taken. These are emergency telephone numbers in most countries for ambulance and medical emergencies. Some countries use more than one number.

Also, at the end of this book, you will find some useful but brief tips on how to deal with a few emergencies (**Apitherapy for first aid in a nutshell**).

112: European Union and other countries. Used in: Akrotiri and Dhekelia (also 999), Åland Islands, Albania, Andorra, Armenia (also 911), Australia, Austria, Azerbaijan, Belarus, Belgium, Bosnia, Bosnia and Herzegovina, Bulgaria, Cameroon, Central African Republic, Clipperton Island, Croatia, Cyprus, Czech　Republic, Democratic Republic of Congo, Denmark, East Timor, Estonia, Egypt (also 911), Falkland Islands (also 999), Faroe Islands, Finland, France, French Guiana, French Polynesia, Gambia, Georgia, Germany, Gibraltar, Greece, Greenland, Guadeloupe, Guernsey, Guinea-Bissau, Herzegovina, Hungary, Iceland, India, Indonesia (also 119), Iran (also 115), Iraq (also 911), Ireland (also 999), Isle of Man, Italy, Jersey (also 999), Kenya (also 999), Kosovo, Kurdistan (also 911), Kuwait, Latvia, Liechtenstein, Lithuania, Luxembourg, Macedonia, Madagascar, Malta, Martinique, Mauritania, Mayotte, Monaco, Montenegro, Nagorno-Karabakh, Netherlands, New Caledonia, Nigeria, Northern Cyprus, Poland, Portugal, Republic of Congo, Reunion, Romania, Russia, Rwanda, Saint Pierre and Miquelon, San Marino, São Tomé and Príncipe, Saudi Arabia (also 911),　Seychelles (also 999), Slovakia, Slovenia, Spain, Sweden, Switzerland, Tajikistan, Togo, Turkey, Turkmenistan, Uganda, Ukraine, United Arab Emirates, United Kingdom (also 999), Uzbekistan, Vanuatu, Vatican City.

911: Canada, United States (North American Numbering Plan). Also in American Samoa, Antarctica, Antigua and Barbuda, Anguilla, Argentina, Aruba, Bahamas (also 919), Barbados, Belize, Bermuda, Bolivia, Bonaire, Botswana, Brazil (also 192), British Virgin Islands (also 999), Cayman Islands, Costa Rica (also 112), Dominican Republic (also 112), Ecuador, Ethiopia, Fiji, Grenada, Guam, Israel (also 101), Jordan (also 112), Liberia, Marshall Islands, Micronesia, Montserrat (also 999), Navassa Island, Palau, Panama, Paraguay, Peru, Philippines, Puerto Rico, Saint Kitts and Nevis, Saint Lucia (also 999), Saint Vincent and the Grenadines, Solomon Islands (also 999),Tonga, Tuvalu, Uruguay, Venezuela, Virgin Islands .

999: United Kingdom and many British territories. Used in: Ascension Island, Bahrain, British Indian Ocean Territory (also 112), Burma, Dominica, Ghana, Guyana, Hong Kong, Kiribati, Macau, Malawi, Malaysia, Oman, Qatar, Saint Helena, Samoa, Sierra Leone, Singapore, South Georgia and the South Sandwich Islands, Sudan, Tristán da Cunha, Zambia, Zimbabwe.

🧰 OTHER NUMBERS FOR MEDICAL EMERGENCIES AND AMBULANCE SERVICES

000: Australia, Christmas Island, Cocos Islands.
066: Mexico (also 911).
14: Algeria.
15: Morocco.
18: Burkina Faso, Cambodia, Chad, Comoros, Djibouti, Gabon, Mali, Niger, Senegal.
102: India, Maldives, Nepal.
103: Abkhazia, Belarus, Kyrgyzstan, Transnistria.
104: Cuba.
105: Mongolia.
110: Bhutan, Jamaica, Sri Lanka, Syria.
111: Nauru, New Zealand, Nigeria, Papua New Guinea.
113: Norway.
114: Mauritius, Tanzania.
115: Angola, Equatorial Guinea, Iran, Mauritius, Pakistan, Surinam, Vietnam.
116: Eritrea, Haiti.
118: Benin, Burundi, Central African Republic, Indonesia.
119: Afghanistan, Cambodia, Japan, North Korea, South Korea, Taiwan.

120: People's Republic of China.
122: Lesotho.
123: Colombia, Egypt.
128: Guatemala.
131: Chile.
132: El Salvador, Nicaragua.
140: Lebanon.
150: Western Sahara.
180: Ivory Coast.
191: Yemen.
192: Brazil.
194: Serbia.
195: Honduras, Laos.
198: Tunisia.
199: Bangladesh.
555: Somalia.
903: Moldova.
912: Curaçao.
933: Swaziland.
990: Trinidad and Tobago.
995: Singapore.
998: Cook Islands.
1515: Libya.
1569: Thailand.
1717: Guinea.
10 177: South Africa.

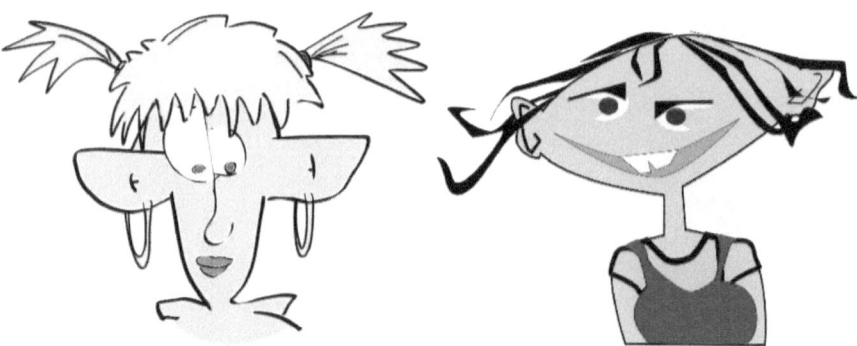

-- APITOXIN MICRO-STINGS INSTEAD OF BOTOX FOR BOOSTING COLLAGEN; PLUS, TOPICAL HONEY, BEE BREAD, AND PROPOLIS ON YOUR FACE; SOME ORAL ROYAL JELLY, DRONE LARVAE, AND POLLEN AS DIET SUPPLEMENTS... NO QUESTION, SOON YOU AND ME WILL BE LIKE BEAUTY QUEENS

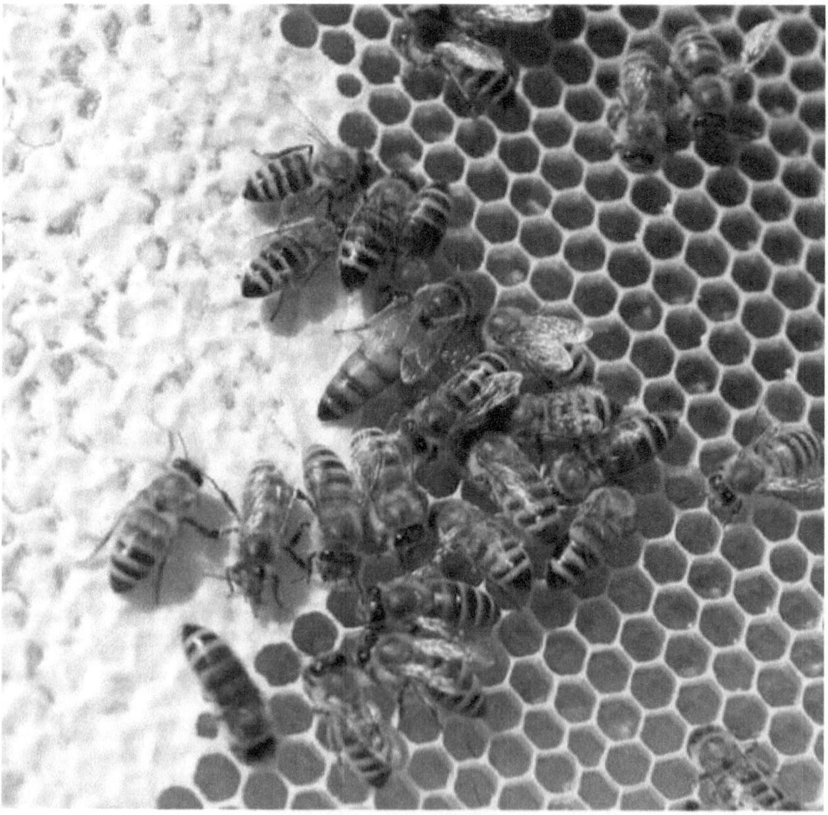

...

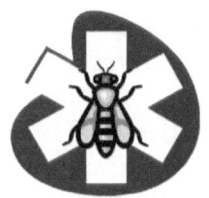

15. ABOUT THE AUTHOR

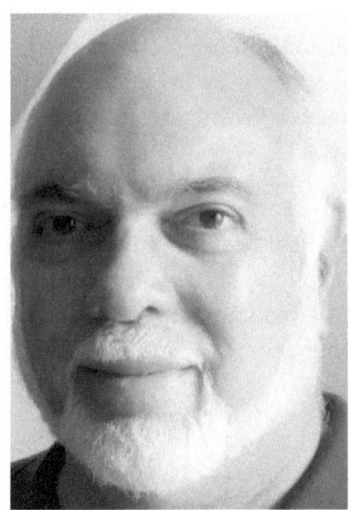

Moisés Asís is a Cuban-American scientist, writer, criminal lawyer, and clinical social worker. He has authored over seventeen books, including essays, plays, and novels, and on subjects such as Apitherapy, Alternative Medicine, Hypnotherapy, Parapsychology, and Judaism, plus over a hundred articles in several languages, in addition to contributions to *Encyclopedia of Cuba: People, History, Culture* (editors Luis Martínez *et al.*), to the anthology *Havana Noir* and *La Havane Noir* (editor Achy Obejas), and to documentary films *Havana Nagila: the Jews* in Cuba (directors Laura Paull & Evan Garelle) and *Cuban America* (director Adelin Gasana). Some book titles are *Propóleo, un valioso producto apícola*; *Propóleo, el oro púrpura de las abejas*; *Tesauro*

parapsicológico de búsqueda informativa; Investigaciones cubanas sobre el propóleo; Los productos de la colmena; Apiterapia para todos; Apiterapia 101 para todos; Apitherapy 101 A-Bee-Z; Parapsicología e hipnosis experimental; Acupuntura y hatha yoga para las disfunciones sexuales; Vulnerables: una historia miamense de amor; Cómo redactar y editar un artículo científico para su publicación (with Carlos R. Pérez); *Hipnosis: teorías, métodos y técnicas* (with Braulio M. Perigod), and *Cuban Miami* (with Robert M. Levine).

Asís received academic degrees (including BSc, JD, PhD, MSW) from Havana University, Open International University for Complementary Medicines, and Florida International University. In 1974, he received two prizes as a playwright in national literary contests by Havana University and by Unión Nacional de Escritores y Artistas de Cuba, and in 1991 his book *Hipnosis: teorías, métodos y técnicas* received an award by Instituto Cubano del Libro and Cuba Academy of Sciences for authoring one of the best 10 scientific and technical books published in Cuba. Asís worked as an information analyst, professor, therapist, clinical social worker and protective investigator (API) in Havana and Miami. In 1993, he immigrated to the United States.

After founding and co-leading the Sociedad Cubana de Hipnosis, he was a board member of the International Apitherapy Healthcare and Bee Acupuncture Association and of the American Apitherapy Society, a founder of Bees for Life – World Apitherapy Network and, at the suggestion of him and other co-founders of Bees for Life, March 30 was designed as the World Apitherapy Day, in honor of Filip Terč (1844 - 1917), Father of Modern Apitherapy.

- Apitherapy101@gmail.com & moisesasis@gmail.com
- Skype.com/moisesasis1
- www.MoisesAsis.com; www.Facebook.com/moises.asis
- www.Linkedin.com/in.moisesasis
- www.Facebook.com/apitherapy101;
  www.Facebook.com/groups/BeesForLifeWorldApitherapy

APITHERAPY FOR FIRST AID IN A NUTSHELL

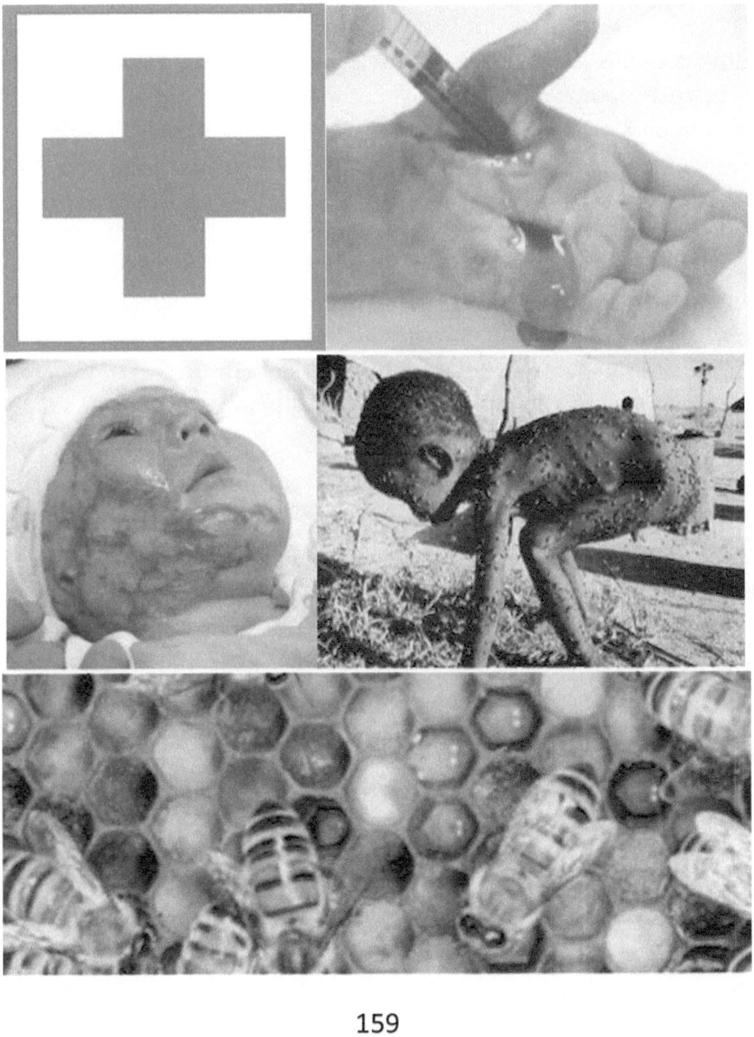

Du, uring the last weeks, while editing and publishing this book, several hurricanes did hit very hard on Texas, Florida (where I live), and other mainland US, and Mexico, Cuba, Puerto Rico, and other Caribbean islands, several earthquakes caused havoc in California, Arizona, Mexico, Japan, New Zealand, Chile, Taiwan, Indonesia, and other regions; epidemics and famine impacted continents; and wars and terrorist massacres damaged many countries. For that reason, I didn't want to leave you without providing before with some useful information in a nutshell you could find, whenever needed, at the end of this book and share it with your friends and family members as the core of non-invasive Apitherapy for emergencies.

Keep handy at home, in your car, and in your worksite or school at least three beehive products that do not deteriorate for years at a room temperature: **honey** (or honeydew honey or both), **propolis** (or géopropolis, honeycomb capping or all), and **bee pollen** (or bee bread or both). Propolis and honey have potentially a shelf life of three-thousand years. You don't need to be a medical doctor or a registered nurse to save someone during a life-threatening emergency before Fire/Rescue and paramedics (see **Chapter 14**) arrive to help with more resources. These are my 10 basic tips for a non-invasive Apitherapy nutshell:

⊕ **AMPUTATIONS, CUTS, LACERATIONS, SCRATCHES, OTHER WOUNDS**: Topical propolis or honey; clean wound with saline and change dressings.

⊕ **ANEMIA, MALNUTRITION, STARVATION:** Oral pollen + honey + water, *ad libitum*. Both pollen and honey are slowly water soluble at room temperature.

⊕ **BACTERIAL, FUNGAL, VIRAL INFECTIONS**: Topical and oral propolis, honey, or both. Oral doses are 2 droppers in a glass of water 3 times a day *ac*.

⊕ **BURNS**: Topical honey or oil propolis. Keep burns covered with dressings.

⊕ **DEHYDRATION, DIARRHEA**: Oral; mix honey (0.5 cup) + orange squeeze or mashed ripe banana (0.5 cup) + kitchen salt (0.1 tsp) + potassium chloride (0.1 tsp) in 4 cups of boiled water. In adults, 3 cups a day; in babies and toddlers, 0.5 cup a day. This formula is adapted from WHO's oral rehydrating solution.

⊕ **INFLAMMATION**: Topical propolis or honey. Checkup causes of edema.

⊕ **INSECT BITES**: Topical propolis extract or honey. Check on anaphylaxis signs.

⊕ **PARASITOSIS**: Oral propolis tincture, 3 droppers in a glass of water 3 times a day one-hour *ac* (before meals). Also, topical propolis applications if needed.

⊕ **RESPIRATORY PROBLEMS**: Vapor inhalation of propolis or honey solutions.

⊕ **SUPERFICIAL PAIN**: Topical propolis extract or tincture. It is anesthetic.